# Sleep Medicine - Asleep or Awake?

*Edited by Tang-Chuan Wang*

Published in London, United Kingdom

Sleep Medicine - Asleep or Awake?
http://dx.doi.org/10.5772/intechopen.104201
Edited by Tang-Chuan Wang

Contributors
Jorge Garza-Ulloa, Magdalena Filcek, Mayank Vats, Michael O. Ogundele, Chinnaiah Yemula, Hani F. Ayyash, Pak Wing Cheng, Yiu Pan Wong, Mohammed Albreiki, Sheikh Saba Naz, Muhammad Muddassar Shafiq, Irina Labunets



First published in London, United Kingdom, 2024 by IntechOpen
IntechOpen is the global imprint of INTECHOPEN LIMITED, registered in England and Wales, registration number: 11086078, 5 Princes Gate Court, London, SW7 2QJ, United Kingdom

British Library Cataloguing-in-Publication Data
A catalogue record for this book is available from the British Library

Additional hard and PDF copies can be obtained from orders@intechopen.com

Sleep Medicine - Asleep or Awake?
Edited by Tang-Chuan Wang
p. cm.
Print ISBN 978-1-83768-556-1
Online ISBN 978-1-83768-557-8
eBook (PDF) ISBN 978-1-83768-558-5

For EU product safety concerns:
IN TECH d.o.o., Prolaz Marije Krucifikse Kozulić 3, 51000 Rijeka, Croatia,
info@intechopen.com or visit our website at intechopen.com.

# Meet the editor

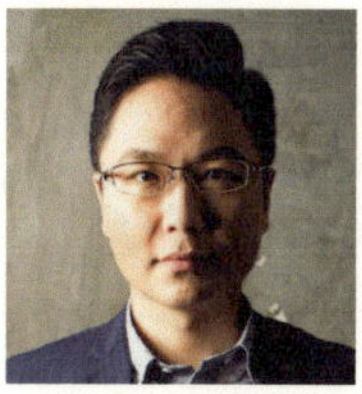

Dr. Tang-Chuan Wang is an excellent otolaryngologist-head and neck surgeon in Taiwan. He is also a research scholar at Harvard Medical School and University of Iowa Hospital, USA. He has extensive experience working at several institutions in the United States, including Stanford University, the University of Pennsylvania, Johns Hopkins University, Boston Children's Hospital, and Massachusetts Eye and Ear. He not only works in clinical and basic medicine but is also expanding into public health in Taiwan. In recent years, Dr. Wang has devoted himself to artificial intelligence and medical innovations. He always says that "in theoretical or practical aspects, no innovation is a step backward." Due to his contribution to biodesign, he was invited to join the executive committee of the Advanced Joint R&D Center in Taiwan.

# Contents

# Preface

Sleep is a kind of naturally recurring state that is associated with muscle relaxation and reduced perception of environmental stimuli, including altered consciousness and relatively inhibited sensory activity. Sleep is, so to speak, one of the most complicated and mysterious things in humans. In fact, opinions on sleep vary across cultures.

From the middle of the 20th century, sleep-related research has provided more and more knowledge and solved many puzzles about sleep-wake functioning. At the same time, there is growing awareness about the significance of sleep and its disorders. The concept of sleep medicine thrived in the second half of the 20th century. The medical profession began showing more interest than previously in primary sleep disorders and the quality of sleep in other conditions. Therefore, sleep medicine is one of the fastest-growing divisions of medicine.

Disorders and disturbances of sleep are wide-ranging and can have significant effects on affected individuals as well as economic consequences for society. For instance, sleep apnea is a kind of sleep disorder characterized by periods of interrupted or shallow breathing during sleep. Sleep apnea has become an essential health issue in the United States. Approximately 22 million Americans suffer from sleep apnea, and 80% of moderate and severe obstructive sleep apnea cases are undiagnosed. Most importantly, sleep medicine should accelerate increased public awareness of sleep disorders and facilitate the consolidation of sleep health into medical care in a responsible fashion. To create a common opinion, we must enfold innovation in sleep medicine.

Since the end of 2019, COVID-19 has made telemedicine more mainstream. This means that clinicians must use wearable or Internet of Things (IoT) devices for disease evaluation and treatment. Personalized data generated by the various monitoring technologies are jointly managed by patients and medical staff. Medical staff will supervise artificial intelligence (AI) algorithms to understand patients' specific conditions and provide the best decision-making and treatment. Thus, the dream of precision medicine will definitely come true in the future.

However, the complex nature of sleep medicine also has led us to re-examine whether existing telemedicine is sufficient to meet higher-level medical needs in theory and practice. In my opinion, scientific testing can help us clarify some problems, but we should not only focus on the cold data but also pay attention to real people. The mysteries between asleep and awake are beyond our imagination. In this book, expert authors provide their own knowledge and experience to provide a comprehensive overview of sleep medicine. The book incorporates updated developments as well as future perspectives in the ever-expanding field of sleep medicine. It is a great reference for medical staff (family doctors, ENTs, neurologists, psychiatrists, psychologists, pulmonologists, registered nurses, and the technologists who perform sleep studies), researchers in sleep medicine, social workers, public health practitioners, experts in science, and even patients themselves.

I appreciate everyone who contributed to the editorial process of this book, including the publishing process manager, commissioning editor, and technical editor at IntechOpen. They made great efforts and their wonderful assistance resulted in the success of this academic work. Finally, I am always full of gratitude for my family, teachers, and colleagues.

**Tang-Chuan Wang (Vincent Wang)**
Chairman of Otolaryngology-Head and Neck Surgery,
China Medical University Hsinchu Hospital,
Taiwan

College of Medicine,
China Medical University,
Taiwan

College of Biomedical Engineering,
China Medical University,
Taiwan

Research Scholar of Harvard Medical School,
MA, USA

Research Scholar of University of Iowa Hospitals and Clinics,
IA, USA

Member of American Academy of Otolaryngology-Head and Neck Surgery
Fellow of the American College of Surgeons

Section 1

# Physiology and Mechanisms – Asleep or Awake

Chapter 1

# Interaction between Melatonin, Sleepiness-Alertness and Body Temperature

*Sheikh Saba Naz, Muhammad Muddassar Shafiq and Mohammed Albreiki*

## Abstract

Circadian rhythms confer a biological clock of all living beings, comprising oscillations in a range of physiological variables, including body temperature and melatonin, that regulate the sleep/wake cycle rhythmically. Both variables have been marked to influence the sleep/wake cycle; even so, the interrelationship among the triad (body temperature, melatonin & sleepiness/alertness) is still unknown. The current literature review is envisioned to examine the contemporary details regarding the interaction between melatonin, body temperature, and sleepiness/alertness. All the included information is procured from the latest review articles, systematic & meta-analytical literature reviews, and original research reports. Findings revealed that melatonin and body temperature collectively contribute to the formation of sleep. An increase in melatonin induces fluctuations in body temperature. Both physiologic variables serve as close indicators of sleepiness/alertness. However, modulating factors such as light, environmental temperature, and timing of melatonin administration (with the circadian clock) may impact the overall outcomes. A significant number of studies are required to infer the underlying processes by which these factors influence the circadian clock.

**Keywords:** Core Body Temperature (CBT), melatonin, sleepiness-alertness, circadian rhythm, light at night (LAN)

## 1. Introduction

Circadian rhythms are a biological trait shared by all organisms, comprised of oscillations in various physiological variables, such as melatonin, body temperature, motor activity, or cortisol production. These rhythms are observable in all members of a given species. Circadian rhythms exist in most human physiological processes, including CBT, heart rate, breathing rate, metabolic rate, activity in many brain regions, hormone release (including cortisol and melatonin), and the sleep-wake cycle. The circadian control of cognitive performance and sleep refers to the almost 24-h cycle of wakefulness and sleepiness. Daytime hours are characterized by heightened alertness and reduced sleepiness, while nocturnal hours display the inverse pattern [1, 2]. These sleep-wake cycles revealed some relationship between body temperature and melatonin levels. Previously, studies have reported a drop in Core Body Temperature (CBT) in the early morning and peek in the evening. In contrast, melatonin levels rise at night and dropped to their nadir in the morning. Alertness refers to the high environmental consciousness and swings in a circadian pattern, having low concentrations during night that are augmented during the day. Studies have suggested dissimilar overlaps between CBT, melatonin, and alertness. Light-induced melatonin suppression has been shown to elevate the scores of alertness. In addition, alterations in CBT can potentially modulate the sleep/wake cycle [1]. These findings suggest some correlation between these three physiologic variables; sleepiness, melatonin, and body temperature. Accordingly, we aim to report the latest information regarding two research questions, (a) Is the alerting effect caused by the cumulative effort of melatonin and body temperature, (b) Does any correlation exist between the three variables?

## 2. Human sleep-wake cycle

A repeating pattern that alternates between waking and sleep is known as the human sleep-wake cycle. The body's intrinsic biological clock (circadian rhythm) and the buildup of sleep pressure (homeostatic factor) are two of the variables that control it. During wakefulness, various neurotransmitter systems promote alertness, while during sleep, different stages like rapid eye movement (REM) and non-rapid eye movement (NREM) facilitate rest and restoration. The NREM and REM sleep stages alternate in roughly 90-minute periods during the course of the night, reiterating the sleep-wake cycle. Understanding and maintaining a healthy sleep-wake cycle is vital for overall well-being and optimal functioning during wakefulness [3–5].

### 2.1 The neurophysiology of sleep and wake

By taking into account the sleep-wake cycle and the underlying neurological processes involved, it is possible to comprehend the neurophysiology of sleep and wakefulness. Rapid eye movement (REM) sleep and non-rapid eye movement (NREM) sleep are the two basic sleep patterns that make up the human sleep cycle. N1, N2, and N3 are the three stages of NREM sleep (**Figure 1**). The N1 stage is the lightest stage, followed by N2 with sleep spindles and K-complexes and N3 with slow, high-amplitude delta waves as the deepest stage. The majority of dreams take place during REM sleep, which is distinguished by rapid eye movement and elevated brain activity. The sleep cycle starts with NREM sleep (N1-N2-N3) and then transitions to REM sleep. This cycle repeats throughout the night, lasting around 90–120 minutes per cycle. NREM sleep is more prominent in the first half of the night, while REM sleep becomes more significant in the later cycles [3, 4, 6].

Neurotransmitter systems play a role in promoting sleep or wakefulness. Sleep-promoting systems involve VLPO neurons, inhibiting wake-promoting systems. Cholinergic neurons promote REM sleep by activating the cortex and paralyzing muscles [7, 8]. Wake-promoting systems use neurotransmitters like acetylcholine and monoamines (serotonin, dopamine, norepinephrine, and histamine). ACh promotes wakefulness through direct projections to the cortex.

A flip-flop circuit model explains how wake- and sleep-promoting mechanisms are mutually inhibited, with the orexin system maintaining sleep-wake behavior [9].

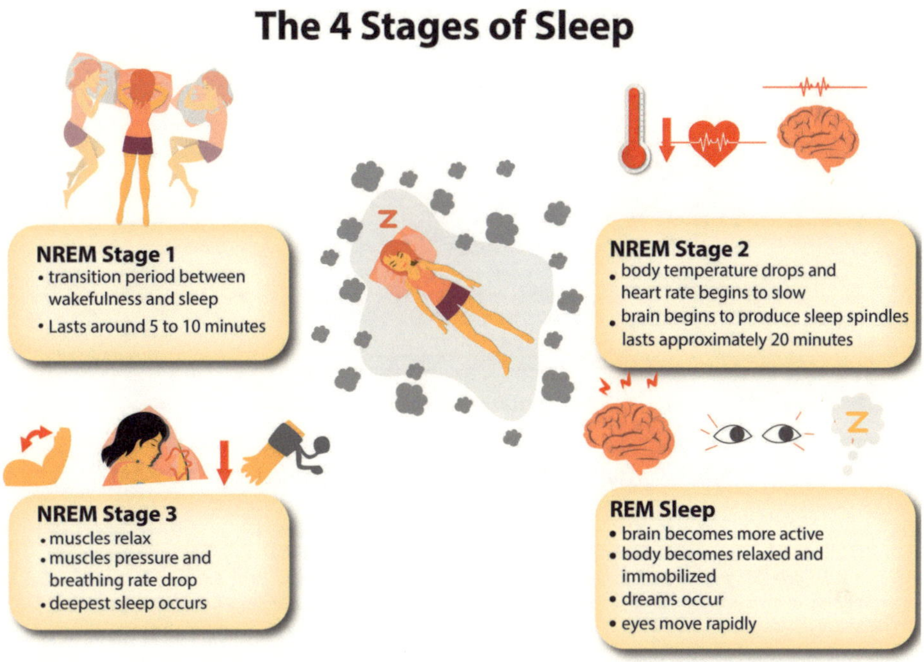


**Figure 1.**
*The four stages of sleep. Figure 1 illustrates the four stages of sleep. The first three stages are known as non-rapid eye movement (NREM) sleep, whereas the fourth stage is known as rapid eye movement (REM) sleep. The brain transitions through four unique stages of sleep several times through the night. Each stage has a unique function and role in maintaining the brain's overall cognitive performance.*

During waking hours, GABA and monoamine neurons are active; however, they are hardly active during NREM sleep and completely silent during REM sleep. The sleep-wake cycle causes changes in neurotransmitter activity. When we are awake, ACh neurons are active, dormant during deep (NREM) sleep, and only partially active during REM sleep. When you are awake, orexin neurons are active, and when you are asleep, they are not [3, 8].

### 2.2 Regulation of sleep-wake cycle: homeostatic and circadian regulation

Two processes, circadian regulation and homeostatic regulation, control the sleep-wake cycle. Process S, or homeostasis, is the process by which sleep pressure builds up during waking and is released during sleep. Adenosine, a substance in the brain, plays a role in increasing sleep pressure, promoting sleepiness. During sleep, adenosine levels decrease, reducing sleep pressure and promoting wakefulness [10].

The body's internal biological clock, also known as process C, is principally managed by the suprachiasmatic nucleus (SCN) in the hypothalamus. The SCN collects data on light exposure and assists in synchronizing the body's internal clock with the external cycle of day and night. The SCN controls how much melatonin the pineal gland secretes. Melatonin levels rise at night, encouraging sleep, and fall in the morning, indicating awakeness [11].

The interaction between homeostatic and circadian regulation is vital for maintaining a healthy sleep-wake cycle (**Figure 2**). The homeostatic process determines the need for sleep based on prior wakefulness, whereas the circadian process

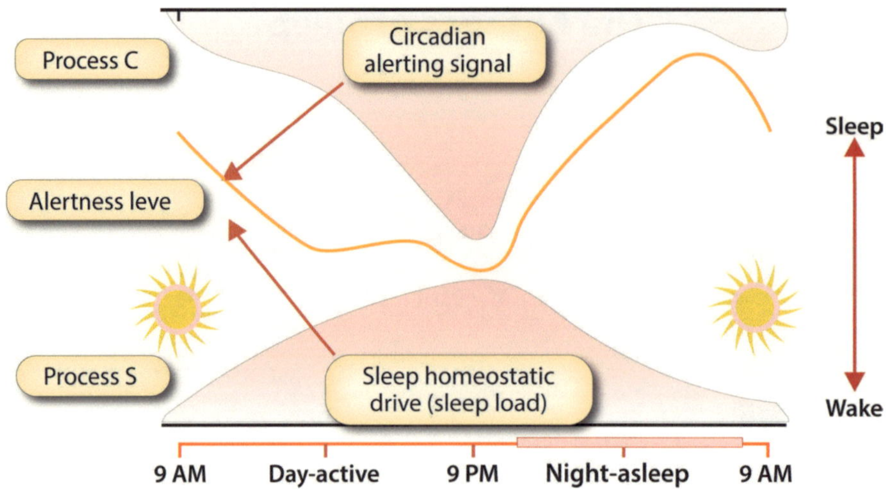


**Figure 2.**
*Homeostatic and circadian regulation of sleep-wake cycle. Figure 2 indicates the two processes that regulate the sleep-wake cycle. Sleepwake cycle is controlled by circadian (Process C) and homeostatic (Process S). The interaction between homeostatic and circadian regulation is important to maintain a healthy sleep-wake cycle.*

uses the light-dark cycle to predict when and how much sleep and wakefulness will occur. Disruptions of these regulatory processes can lead to sleep disorders and irregular sleep patterns [12].

## 3. Sleepiness and alertness; description, definition, and measure

Sleep is an elementary component of mammalian homeostatic mechanisms. The homeostatic regulation of sleep is fundamentally processed by the physiology of the circadian clock (sleep/wake cycle). Sleepiness and alertness are entirely distinct constructs. Sleepiness can be illustrated as a proclivity to fall asleep. It is a homeostatic measure characterized by a perpetual sleep-wake cycle in the absence of motivational and affective factors and can be modulated by circadian factors and sleep debt. However, alertness is the propensity of the brain to respond optimally to internal and external stimuli, and it may vary erratically. Neurophysiological substrates serve as a potential mediator that governs motivation, affect, and cognitive potential required for alertness [1].

An experience of feeling sleepy or alert is driven by perplexed interactions of neurophysiological pathways that exhibit dissimilar overlaps in different states of consciousness, impairment, and illness and can be influenced by numerous factors (external stimuli or stressors) [9]. These pathways can be modulated by melatonin, dopamine, hypocretin/orexin, serotonin, and norepinephrine. These neurohormones and neurotransmitters are also involved in the control of appetite, attention, fight-or-flight, and motivation [1, 9].

With time, various methods have been devised to quantify sleepiness or alertness. Multiple sleep latency tests (MSLT) can determine excessive daytime sleepiness or weakened alertness under controlled conditions [13]. The maintenance of the Wakefulness test is another objective test to ascertain a person's potential to stay awake during a defined period. It also helps to evaluate the success rate of the patient's treatment plan [14]. Other alternatives include patient self-scoring questionnaires, namely ESS (Epworth sleepiness scale; 24 points), an instant KSS (Karolinska Sleepiness Scale; 9 points), THAT (50-points), ZOGIMA-A (50 points) and SSS (Stanford sleepiness scale; 7 points). ESS is instrumental in subjectively examining sleepiness [15]. The ZOGIMA-A is an alertness questionnaire that presents a level of alertness in the reflection of hypothetical scenarios (that may manipulate the subject's alertness) and a percentage rating scale of other activities (where alertness is required) [16]. Based on 50 points, the THAT questionnaire facilitates the retrospective investigation of the energy and concentration of the subject [17]. SSS helps in the estimation of subjective sleepiness [18].

### 3.1 Circadian rhythm and human sleepiness-alertness

The body's internal clock comprises 24-h circadian rhythm (CR) cycles that work in the background to carry out vital processes and functions. These rhythms are recorded oscillations influenced by physiological variables, such as melatonin, body temperature, cortisol secretion, and motor activities. The sleep-wake cycle is one of the most significant and well-known circadian rhythms [19].

Alteration in physiological variables can result in acute variations in these oscillations. For instance, when a mammal runs spontaneously to avoid a predator, the intense exercise boosts body temperature for a few minutes before the effect wears off and the temperature returns to its normal circadian range. These fleeting physiologic changes obscure circadian rhythms. The 24-h cycles (circadian rhythms) of sleepiness and alertness substantially influence cognitive performance and sleep. High alertness exists at daytime hours, and more sleepiness is observed at night [20].

According to the Posner and Rafal neuropsychological model, alertness constitutes four elements: sustained attention, selective attention, tonic alertness, and phasic alertness [21]. Sustained attention pertains to responding efficiently to an extended period (minutes to hours). Selective attention corresponds to the precise and selective response to every stimulus. Tonic alertness is an accustomed response to the environment induced by generic phenomena at any time. Phasic alertness refers to the response that generates following a warning signal, for example, a change of environment. The brain systems that chiefly contribute to upholding the alertness-linked circadian rhythms include the prefrontal, reticular, and parietal systems. The results of nearly all tests and tasks are compromised when attention-associated components are impacted by brain injury or any other disorder [21, 22].

The estimation of cognitive performance (alertness), regulated by the variations of circadian rhythms, can be performed by simple reaction or vigilance tasks. With reference to tonic and phasic alertness, Psychomotor Vigilance Test measured cognitive performance by modulating homeostatic and circadian rhythms, such as persistent routine, time of day, and forced asynchronism [23]. Reports corroborated an increase in reaction time, with lower response latency during the day and higher response latency at night. The frequency of lapses (omissions or responses with delayed reaction times) increased in the restive period and experienced circadian variations, with fewer lapses during the day and more at night [24, 25]. Variations in homeostatic (time awake) and circadian (time of day) cycles have remarkably influenced selective attention scores under the constant routine protocol. On providing a short interval among two stimuli (T1 and T2), progressive response latency was observed with the second stimuli (T2; lag 2, 200 ms) and the successive independent stimulus (T2; lag 8800 ms) [26]. Assessment of sustained attention can be carried out by measuring three indices: stability in performance efficiency, time on task performance, and short-term stability. These variables can be examined by analyzing the variability of correct responses throughout the task. High stability can be depicted when the responses exhibit less variability. Accordingly, high attention scores were recorded during the day and less at night [27]. These investigations presented a direct relationship between time awake and the decline in alertness. Also, the dual task and task-switching performance was retarded due to sleep deprivation [2].

The impaired mechanisms of sleep generation may induce the propensity of acquiring SCRD (sleep and circadian rhythm disruption) disorder, ensued by comorbidity or lack of opportunity to sleep. The SCRD corresponds to the lack of optimal sleep duration, poor sleep quality, and improper sleep patterns. There are 83 types of sleep disorders listed in the ICSD (International Classification of Sleep Disorders), 3rd edition. The disruption of circadian rhythms eventuates in conditions that include Free-running sleep disorder (FRSD), Delayed sleep phase disorder (DSPD), Advanced sleep phase disorder (ASPD), Fragmented sleep disorder (FSD), and Insomnia. ASPD is characterized by falling asleep in the evening and trouble sleeping in the early morning. The DSPD appertains to the onset and offset of ≥3 h. sleep latency. FRSD is attributed to progressive sleep latency each day. FSD is observed in patients with complete loss of circadian clock. The term "insomnia" refers to a condition where a person has trouble falling or staying asleep [28].

## 4. Light and human sleepiness-alertness

### 4.1 Effect of LAN on alertness

Light exhibits acute alerting effects that can potentially influence the performance of night-shift workers. From a circadian standpoint, one of the possible underlying mechanisms is the suppression of melatonin ensued by high-intensity light exposure. However, the effects of light cannot be exacted as numerous factors, such as endogenous circadian phase, prior environmental light exposure, and duration of prior wakeful period, significantly affect the overall outcomes [29]. The majority of the studies have analyzed the impact during the night. To apprehend the correlation between light exposure and circadian and homoeostatic functioning, Chellapa et al. have reported a dramatic upsurge of subjective alertness and reduction in the objective markers of sleepiness (e.g. movement of the eye), even under high sleep pressure [30].

Some studies have additionally credited the attenuation of SCN (suprachiasmatic nucleus) depending on mechanisms caused by melatonin. It may regulate and stimulate the arousal of cortical and behavioral states at certain points in circadian cycles. A study aimed to determine the comparative influence of alertness for three different light conditions; continuous bright light, intermittent bright light (alternative exposure of dim light and bright light), and dim light with a 3-h exposure, rendered insignificant differences between continuous and intermittent bright light exposure; however, KSS scores were remarkably lower in intermittent light conditions than in dim light conditions. Over time, a progressive decline of subjective alertness was observed among all exposures; however, the objective alertness was considerably higher in the cohort of intermittent exposure compared to the subjects that experienced dim light conditions. In comparison with dim light conditions, intermittent and continuous light exposures scored low for total sleep time and sleep efficiency, but the sleep pattern was marginally affected [31]. Similarly, subjective alertness was significantly lower during dim light and/or melatonin administration in comparison to bright light exposure [32]. Contrarily, some studies did not evidence any light-inducing alerting effects (AE) or melatonin suppression during the day or night. Thus, the presence of additional mechanistic activities can be a plausible explanation for this phenomenon. Light intensity is significant for ideal synchronization of the two variables (sleepiness or alertness), as more than 1000 lux polychromic light may escalate AE, irrespective of timing (day or night). It transposes the scientists to secondary analysis, i.e. Calculation of the Light Intensity Threshold that renders AE [31].

### 4.2 Effect of light intensity/wavelength on alertness

Ocular light exposure poses adverse effects on the human circadian clock. In particular, specific light intensities (wavelengths) can potentially synchronize (entrain) endogenous circadian rhythms to the 24-h day and eventuate in a variable alerting effect. Sunde et al. investigated the comparative alerting effect of a 455 nm- short wavelength narrow bandwidth light and 625 nm- long-wavelength narrow bandwidth light, subjected with a similar photon density (~2.8 × 1014 photons/$cm^2$/s) throughout the nocturnal shift. With long wavelengths, the subject's sleepiness and efficient task performance were more critically influenced than with the subjects exposed to shorter wavelengths. In contrast to long-wavelength light exposed subjects, Psychomotor Vigilance Task (PVT) test displayed more attentive scores in short-wavelength light, characterized by the quick response time, quick response time in the optimal range, and less attentional lapses. In addition, the inception of melatonin was more phase delayed in short-wavelength light than in long-wavelength light. It infers that alertness and performance can be improved with short-wavelength narrow-band light [33]. Blue light (shorter wavelength; 450–495 nm) manifested increased alertness and reaction latency in slightly more than two third of the studies, while decreased sleep efficacy and increased sleep latency among half and slightly less than half of the studies, respectively [34]. This research is consistent with the CDC report regarding the impact of blue light on sleep. Among blue, white, red, and yellow, blue strongly influence the sensitive period (sleep) featured by the inability to fall asleep and stay asleep [35]. Lin et al. dug more to apprehend the impact (AE) from short wavelength on four different frequency bins; theta alpha (5–9 Hz), lower alpha (8–9 Hz), higher alpha (11–13 Hz), and beta (13–30 Hz). Significant associations were established at theta alpha and beta ranges; however, lower alpha and higher alpha presented an insignificant effect. A descriptive posthoc comparison of the beta range accentuated a significant difference between 80 lux and 160 lux, 40 lux and 160 lux, and Dim and 160 lux blue lights. However, a lower AE was observed at 40 lux and 160 lux blue lights. The beta range (160 lux) revealed a remarkable difference compared to the three lighting conditions. According to a KSS score, Subjective sleepiness was considerably reduced in 160 lux conditions than in dim light conditions, affirming a high alerting effect [36]. These findings delineate that short wavelengths, except for a few frequency bins, induce less alertness than longer wavelengths.

## 5. Body temperature and sleep

### 5.1 Physiological regulation of body temperature

Thermoregulation is a term that refers to the maintenance of body temperature. Two types of systems mainly regulate the body temperature: physiological and behavioral. Heat is produced or lost by physiological effectors, which are mostly autonomic and involuntary. The main physiological reactions to cold exposure involve heat production by skeletal muscle contractions, brown adipose tissue (BAT) thermogenesis, and the vasoconstriction (constriction of blood vessels), that inhibits heat loss. However, exposure to warmth induces a set of thermoregulatory autonomic mechanisms, such as sweating (water evaporation) mediated heat loss, repression of thermogenesis, and vasodilation (blood vessels dilation). Different species employ distinct mechanisms to attain similar physiologic effect. For instance, humans utilize sweating to relieve ancillary heat, rodents spread saliva on their fur, and dogs perform panting. Despite these apparent differences, it is believed that a shared set of neuronal substrates that are conserved across mammalian species controls the major physiologic responses [37–39].

Sensory neurons that measure body temperature are the main input source for the thermoregulatory system. Most of these sensory neurons have axons that extend outside their cell bodies to measure the temperature of vital thermoregulatory tissues (e.g. spinal cord, the skin, and abdominal viscera). Also, the temperature of the hypothalamus is sensed and measured by a different set of sensory neurons present in the brain itself.

The thermoregulatory system maintains the temperature set point, which can be modulated by internal and external influencers. They mainly reflect interactions with other physiologic systems. For instance, a controlled body temperature increases (fever) in response to infection. Sleep is another physiological process that imparts modification in and is influenced by the thermoregulatory system. The temperature decline of the body is closely related to sleep onset. During sleep, RED (Rapid Eye Moment) accompanies a near-total inhibition of thermoregulatory responses in most of the species. Long durations and CR-induced diurnal-thermal fluctuations overlay the sleep effects. Neuronal circuits (located in the anterior hypothalamus) control the triad (circadian rhythms, sleep, and body temperature), but the interrelationship of these neural circuits is yet to determine [38, 39].

### 5.2 Body temperature variation with the sleep-wake cycle

Sleep is triggered by a temporal variation in the brain and core body, regulated by a conserved circadian rhythm; however, dissociation from this phenomenon is referred to as Insomnia. A plunge of sleepiness, reduced rapid eye moment and latency of sleep are the stereotypical effects of heat or cold exposure. The environmental influence of temperature induces the thermoregulatory mechanisms linked to sleep. The sleep stages are also affected by the type of bedding or clothing. Heavy clothing and bedding impart high heat exposure, resulting in increased wakefulness, sleep latency, and decreased rapid eye moment. Exposure to humid heat aggravates sleep by escalating thermal load. Contrastingly, cold exposure, with appropriate clothing and bedding conditions, revealed an insignificant impact on the sleep cycle; even so, cold exposure profoundly impacts autonomic responses of the heart without modulating subjective sensations [40–42]. In another study, temperature variation was substantially observed in the morning (post-wakeup) and the evening (pre-sleep). In particular, a transitory state was noted from 6:00 to 10:00 (early to mid-morning) and 18;00 to 22:00 (evening). These transitions are attributed to heat gain in the morning (CBT rises) and loss of heat in the evening (CBT drops). In addition, light considerably contributes to the modulation of thermo-physiological responses in the morning and evening.

In contrast, no change was observed in the core body and distal skin temperature during the afternoon. These results establish a positive association between cold temperatures to increase sleep propensity, whereas hot and humid temperatures may result in less and delayed sleep induction. Furthermore, transitory periods are fundamental in thermo-physiological variations. The thermo-physiological variations can be inferred by collecting 24 h data, with the admissible error rate from inter-individual and exogenous differences, such as irregular eating and sleeping patterns, irregular patterns of light exposures, and jetlag [43].

### 5.3 Regulation of body temperature and sleep

Mammals possess a conspicuous thermal preference for sleep, such as a thermo-neutral environment (27–30°C) and minimal expenditure of energy. These behaviors drive the thermal decline of the circadian cycle (following light and dark cycles) to stimulate sleep. The thermoregulatory mechanisms and sleep are coherently connected with the neural circuits. These circuits employ the warmth to gate sleep, with a simultaneous elevation of circadian cooling of the body to generate the first non-rapid eye moment (NREM). Similar neurons directly connect the NREM initiation to decrease the body temperature [44, 45]. This phenomenon explains the transitional mechanisms that convert wakefulness to NREM sleep, followed by an instant reduction of brain temperature and a subsequent Rapid Eye Moment (REM). A rewarming effect is induced to reverse the phenomenon. NREM is originated in the preoptic hypothalamus (PO) and is activated by warm stimuli. The NREM sleep-inducing brain cooling mechanism and the coordination of circadian rhythm to regulate core temperature are significant to generate efficient sleep [44, 46].

Sleep-stimulating neurons exist all around the brain. It may integrate the autonomous and behavioral nervous systems that cumulatively govern the circadian and homeostatic sleep drive. For instance, the suppression of VTA (ventral tegmental area)-dopamine neurons produces an encouraging effect for sleep initiation [47]. The behavioral, circadian, homeostatic, and autonomic systems generate a cumulative input to gate sleep.

Inefficient thermal systems may modulate the energy-consuming mechanisms and the urge to consume food. Thus, it may solely influence the sleep networks. After a meal, leptin is released by adipocytes. This hormone inhibits hunger and function through multi-stream procedures in the hypothalamic nucleus. In this region, leptin restricts the expression of Neuropeptide Y (NPY), expressing Agouti-related protein (AgRP). The activity of these neurons is repressed to promote sleep. Leptin receptors are also present in the PO hypothalamus. The leptin receptors residing on PO glutamatergic neurons get excited upon arousal of ambient temperature [47, 48].

Consequently, inhibited thermogenesis results in less food consumption and reduced energy dissipation. According to a recent analysis, circulatory leptin and insulin inhibit the AgRP neurons. AgRP neurons are referred to as "hunger sensors" because they can detect energy input. However, Proopiomelanocortin (POMC) neurons exhibit an opposite mode of action. AgRP activates food-seeking behavior by compromising sleep. However, in the case of food deprivation, AgRPs are repressed to secure sleep at the expense of food; sleep deprivation radically alters the energy balance and thermoregulatory mechanisms [44, 49]. From a rat study, the selective REM and chronic sleep deprivation led to detrimental physiological effects and subsequent death [50]. Earlier, high metabolic activity was observed, accompanied by high food consumption and an ascension in body temperature. Then, a sudden drop in temperature ensued in hypothermic conditions among rats [51]. Over time, deepened sleep deprivation results in the progressive rise of body temperature. This data reveals that a range of thermoregulatory mediators, either directly or indirectly, plays a significant part in the stimulation of sleep, depending upon different environmental and bodily conditions [44].

### 5.4 Regulation of body temperature by SCN

The suprachiasmatic nucleus (SCN), which is controlled by the circadian rhythm, is essential in controlling body temperature. The SCN receives information from the eyes regarding the light-dark cycle, which aids in synchronizing the body's internal clock with the outside world. Timing the changes in body temperature is one of its primary duties (**Figure 3**).

Normally, body temperature follows a circadian rhythm, with a decrease at night and an increase during the day. The SCN orchestrates this rhythm by initiating cooling processes during the evening and nighttime. This drop in temperature promotes sleep onset and facilitates restorative sleep. Hormones and neurotransmitters, such as melatonin, are released by the SCN to influence thermoregulation [3, 52].

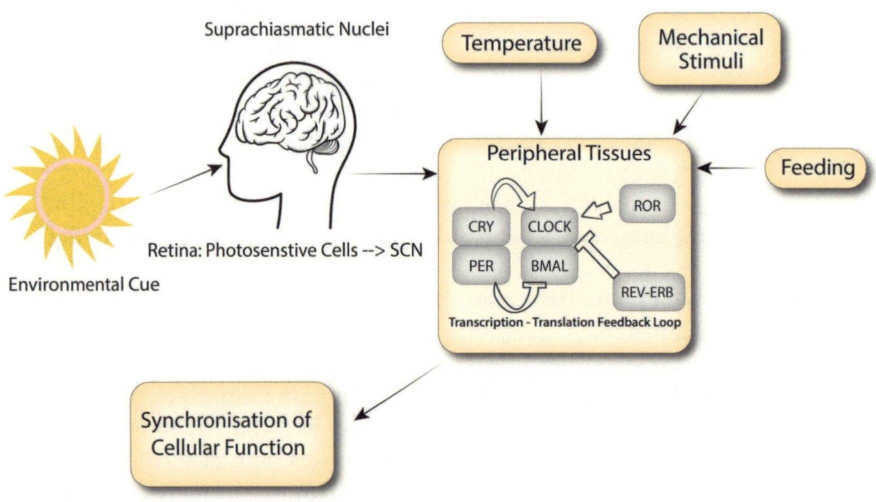


**Figure 3.**
*Schematic summary of circadian synchronization. Figure 3 demonstrates the summary of circadian synchronization. The photic zeitgeber entertains the central clock, which in turn regulates the peripheral clock. The non-photic zeitgebers such as mechanical stimuli, temperature, and feeding mainly entertain the peripheral clock.*

In the morning and throughout the day, as light exposure increases, the SCN triggers the warming process, leading to a rise in body temperature. This promotes wakefulness and alertness. Hormones and neurotransmitters, like cortisol, are released to support wakefulness.

The SCN's regulation of body temperature involves complex interactions with other brain regions and physiological systems. It communicates with areas responsible for thermoregulation, such as the hypothalamus, to coordinate temperature changes throughout the body [12, 52]. Disruptions to the SCN's regulation of body temperature can occur due to factors like jet lag, shift work, or sleep disorders. These disruptions can affect the adjustment to new time zones, disrupt the body's temperature rhythm, and contribute to sleep disturbances.

### 5.5 Circadian rhythm of human body temperature

Human body temperature exhibits a circadian rhythm characterized by 0.8–1°C oscillation that fluctuates between a nocturnal minimum and a diurnal maximum. The circadian rhythms are governed by the hypothalamic SCN (chief thermoregulatory hub in animals) that deploys the TRPs (transient receptor potential; family of ion channels) to detect temperature. Thermal TRPs are frequently expressed in sensory neurons and are triggered at specific temperature thresholds. The subtype TRPV3 detects heat, while the subtype TRPM8 sense cold. Consequently, pre-entering the hypothalamus, thermal information from the integumentary surface, core organs, peripheral tissues, and the neuronal axis itself is combined at multiple levels. The hypothalamic thermoregulatory center receives a rhythmic input from hypothalamus to synchronize with CRBT (Circadian Rhythm of Body Temperature) [53]. Nam et al. demonstrated that the synthesis and metabolism of brown adipose tissue serve as a critical organ for thermal regulation and are coordinated by the circadian clock [54]. Additionally, the seasons could be a possible source of body temperature variation. A large-scale investigation demonstrated that the human circadian cycle exhibits a temperature difference of ~0.2°C between winters and summers. These ambient effects reside within the thermo-tolerable ranges [55]. The circadian system endures significant changes during an individual's lifetime, notably during early old age and in early ontogenetic development. Some reports are evident that daily temperature level and amplitude decrease with age. These changes might be induced due to inefficient intrinsic thermoregulatory mechanisms. They could also be linked to chronic diseases, a sedentary lifestyle or medications and may influence other circadian functions [56]. Furthermore, gender is another substantial factor mainly influenced by sexual hormones. During ovulation, a 0.25–0.5°C rise in body temperature is commonly observed in females. In the luteal phase, the average daily body temperature rises by nearly 0.4°C compared to the pre-ovulatory follicular phase. It is unprecedented that the menstrual event can potentially alter the CRBT [57]. However, progesterone reduces the amplitude and possibly delays the phase of the circadian rhythm in the luteal phase, than in the follicular phase, hence blunting the drop in nocturnal temperature. An altered thermal CR can also result from a disturbed environment, sickness, ambient temperature, sleep, meals, physical activity, or medicines. Night workers display significant CR anomalies including thermal dysregulation of the body, which persists even after retirement [58].

## 5.6 Acute light effects on body temperature

### *5.6.1 The direct impact of LAN on body temperature*

Our circadian temperature is synchronized with the ambient light-dark cycle through the influence of light. Hence, circadian photoentrainment may potentially alter human thermal responses. From 15 studies, evening bright light exposure revealed less decline of CBT compared to dim light conditions. Moreover, a smaller decrease in CBT (0.2°C) was observed with shorter wavelengths than with longer wavelengths [59]. Among 15, two studies documented a decreased melatonin concentration with increased CBT [60, 61]. Two studies reported that longer wavelengths could not reduce CBT in the evening [60, 62]. It advocates the intercedence of pRGCs (photosensitive retinal ganglion cells) that impedes the light induced-natural CBT decline during the night, similar to the CR-phase shifting, where the impact is especially vulnerable to the shorter wavelengths [63]. In another study, 100-lux light exposure was relatable to 10-lux light exposure [63]. Regarding morning exposures, an earlier rise of CBT was observed (0.1°C, by the end of the morning, 0.2°C; during the afternoon, 0.1°C; evening), post bright light exposure in the morning.

Concerning Skin temperature (ST), evening exposure to intense light elevated the mean ST by 1.0°C, compared to light exposure with <50 lux intensity. In contrast, the ST of the foot was approximately −2.0°C lower when exposed to bright light exposure in the evening compared to dim light [64, 65]. Evening's bright light could be the contributing factor that increases Proximal Skin Temperature (PROX-ST) and decreases Distal Skin Temperature (DIST-ST). Regarding DPG (distal to proximal SKT gradient), it was discovered that monochromatic light at both 460 and 550 nm prevents the nighttime temperature decline by 0.7°C. Similar effects on DPG were observed following the bright light exposure in the evening and throughout the night [60, 66]. Melatonin concentration appeared to be reduced at night post-bright light exposure. Evening reduction of melatonin led to an increase in proximal temperatures, a decrease in distal temperatures, and a greater DPG [59].

The impact of Sweat (SW) was analyzed under three experiments. No significant difference was noticed between the effects of blue and red light on SW. However, the bright light exposure in the morning resulted in sweating at −0.1°C, indicating a lower CBT value than in dim light. Sweating may have initiated at the same time and with a similar ST from both light exposures, although bright light exposure reflected lower CBT and no significant difference in ST was observed throughout both exposures. However, bright light exposure revealed lower CBT levels than in dim light [67, 68]. In summary, these findings indicate that evening bright light exposure suppresses melatonin, CBT, and proximal ST while decreasing distal ST. Light exposure in the morning causes an earlier rise in CBT and a quicker drop in melatonin levels. Studies conducted in the afternoon found no correlation between light exposure and CBT or SKT. These results suggest that the influence of bright light on DPG, SKT, and CBT varies with the time of day, the intensity, and the photo-spectral composition. However, future studies are required to examine the persistence of these effects independent from CR-linked phase alteration or melatonin suppression [59].

*5.6.2 Hypothermic effect of melatonin on core temperature*

Melatonin (MLT), a result of pineal gland secretion, significantly contribute in the human circadian clock and exhibits hypothermic and soporific effects. The spike in nocturnal melatonin levels translates into the nadir of CBT. The fact that exogenous MLT exhibits hypothermic qualities are well-documented, although the mechanisms behind this phenomenon is still under investigation. Scientists have observed that MLT promotes peripheral vasodilation without affecting heart rate or cerebral blood flow, suggesting that melatonin operates on peripheral vascular receptors [69].

Likewise, Cook et al. observed that MLT enhanced forearm blood flow and reduced renal blood flow, though cerebral blood flow remained unchanged. These changes in vascular blood flow reflect that heat loss processes primarily drive the hypothermic effects of MLT. The average decrease in CBT after receiving melatonin was calculated to be 0.21°C (0.18–0.24°C) [70]. Cagnacci et al. showed that daytime melatonin administration ensured a quick increase (within 20 minutes) in endogenous MLT and a concurrent reduction in CBT [71]. According to Van den Heuvel et al., MLT suppresses morning CBT for at least 1–2 h after plasma melatonin levels recover to regular daytime values [72]. Researchers discovered that low-dose melatonin injections prevented the body's typical daytime rise in core temperature for *30–90 minutes. Satoh and Mishima observed that the exogenous melatonin's hypothermic effect existed for ~3 h. The extent of suppression was significantly associated with endogenous melatonin levels. Thus, a logarithmic pattern of dose-response was established between MLT doses and their hypothermic effect. A 5-mg dosage of MLT resulted in a *0.2 C drop in body temperature. Higher dosages did not remarkably augment this hypothermic effect; however, they possibly manifest soporific side effects [69, 73].

## 6. Interaction between melatonin, sleepiness-alertness, and body temperature

The relationship of the triad (melatonin, sleepiness/alertness, body temperature) establishes a complex pattern. MLT is chiefly synthesized in the pineal gland, and SCN controls its release. MLT theoretically mediates the communication between the products of the circadian pacemaker and the sleep-wake cycle system. Observed nocturnal periods of sleep inclination under an ultrashort sleep-wake cycle appears to coincide with an increase in melatonin release close to the habitual bedtime. Another study from this review evinced a strong relationship between melatonin suppression with increased alertness, circadian phase shifting, and nocturnal decline [1]. In 2006, blue light (460 nm) exposure enormously suppressed melatonin, accompanied by the decline of subjective sleepiness and increased cognitive performance. In the same year, Lockley et al. established an inverse proportionality between melatonin suppression and arousal of alertness [74]. Contrastingly, Lin et al. expressed a pronounced stimulatory effect of red light for the arousal of alertness while conserving melatonin levels [36]. These studies are consistent with Plitnick et al. and Figueiro et al., where red light elicited subjective alertness, but not at the expense of melatonin [75, 76]. Likewise, Foster RG signified melatonin as a biological marker of the dark that is regulated by a light-inducing mechanism. It has the potential to reduce sleep latency and improve sleep duration. Still, melatonin-deprived individuals (for instance, tetraplegic individuals, pinealectomized patients, and people on beta-blockers) exhibit a rhythmic sleep/wake cycle with marginal alteration [28]. These studies corroborated that melatonin possibly establishes a close association with sleep-inducing mechanisms; however, some additional factors have also facilitated sleep generation.

While exploring coupling mechanisms between the circadian pacemaker and sleep, one alternate theory argues that an indirect influence of melatonin on the sleep-wake cycle mediated by temperature may be crucial, as melatonin has a substantial effect on the temperature rhythm [30]. This theory was formerly evidenced in 2006, where post two hours of melatonin administration revealed a decline of PROX-ST (skin temperature of stomach, thigh, forehead, and infra-clavicular skin regions), and an upsurge of DIST-ST (skin temperature of hand and feet) [77]. A laboratory experiment envisioned to examine the kinetics of melatonin.

degradation plotted a graph between temperatures; 60, 70, 80, and 90°C against the function of time. From a function-of-time standpoint, the highest degradation of melatonin was observed at maximum temperature. In addition, the lowest melatonin levels were recorded in the presence of light at (RT) room temperature. Due to the increased kinetic energy of the reactant molecules, the pace of a reaction typically increases with temperature [78]. In 2019, a study orchestrated the correlational attributes of melatonin, sleepiness/alertness, and temperature. Following melatonin ingestion, subjective sleepiness and DSTL-ST were elicited. On light exposure and post-melatonin administration, PROX-ST increased, and DIST-ST decreased, while alertness scores remained unaffected [79].

Bright light exposure following MLT administration did not alter subjective or alertness scores. Even so, body and PROX-ST increased while DIST-ST decreased. Light exposure unremarkably affects these parameters in the placebo condition. These results confirm a significant association of melatonin in sleep induction, while the thermal association of melatonin still requires additional inquiry. A meta-analysis of 30 datasets revealed a mean drop of 0.21C at 5 mg exogenous melatonin. High soporific effects were recorded at >5 mg dose, though no further temperature decline was observed [69]. With a 5 mg dose, an increase in subjective sleepiness and DSTL-ST was noticed. Following light exposure, DSTL-ST was decreased, and PROX_ST was increased [1]. In a different study, light-induced melatonin declines conferred timing-related thermal fluctuations, where light exposure in the evening revealed a delayed reduction of CBT and decelerated the rise of DST-ST, a morning exposure resulted in a rapid decrease of melatonin and subsequent increase of CBT [59]. An investigation devoid of melatonin accentuated NREM initiation at the steepest rate of decline in body temperature (**Figure 4**) [44].

Conclusively, sleep generation is a cumulative effort of melatonin and body temperature. Also, the rise of melatonin revealed a fluctuation in body temperature. High amounts of MLT correspond to a drop in CBT and PROX-ST, and a rise in DIST-ST. However, the influence of light inhibits the MLT release and subsequently prevents the decline of temperature. Both physiologic variables (body temperature and MLT) serve as close indicators of sleepiness/alertness. However, modulating factors such as light, environmental temperature, and timing of melatonin administration (with reference to the circadian clock) may alter the overall outcomes. Studies constituting large sample sizes are required to infer the underlying mechanisms through which these factors may modulate the circadian clock (**Table 1**).

*DOI: http://dx.doi.org/10.5772/intechopen.112249*

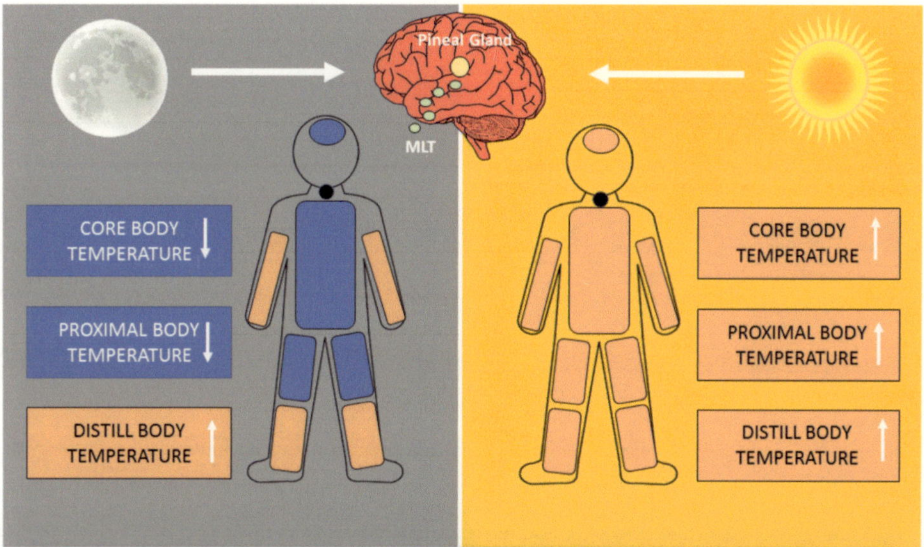


***Figure 4. Comparative influence of light in melatonin synthesis and temperature modulation.***
At night, pineal gland synthesize high amounts of melatonin that causes the drop of CBT and PROX-ST, and increases the DIST-ST. During the day, bright light exposure inhibits the synthesis of melatonin, and no drop of temperature is observed.

**Figure 4.**
*Comparative influence of light in melatonin synthesis and temperature modulation. At night, pineal gland synthesizes high amounts of melatonin that cause the drop of CBT and PROXST and increases the DIST-ST. During the day, bright light exposure inhibits the synthesis of melatonin, and no drop in temperature is observed.*

| Author | Article type | Study year | Studies included/ no. of subjects | Melatonin (MLT) | Sleepiness (S) | Body temperature effect € |
|---|---|---|---|---|---|---|
| Marrin et al. [17] | Review Article | 2013 | 30/193 | 5 mg MLT ▲ | Unknown (Un) | CBT ▼ |
| | | | | >5 mg MLT ▲ | S ▲ | No effect |
| te Kulve et al. [16] | Review Article | 2016 | 48/Un | MLT ▼ | — | CBT ▲ |
| Hardling et al. [20] | Review Article | 2019 | ~160/Un | — | S ▲ | CBT ▼ |
| Lok R. et al. [1] | Research Article | 2019 | 10 subjects | 5 mg MLT ▲ | S ▲ | DSTL-ST ▲ |
| | | | | | | PROX-ST ▼ |
| Krauchi et al. [18] | Research Article | 2006 | 11 subjects | 5 mg MLT ▲ | S ▲ | DSTL-ST ▲ |
| | | | | | | PROX-ST ▼ |

**Table 1.**
*Interplay of melatonin, sleepiness, and body temperature. Table 1 illustrates the collection of research articles demonstrating the interaction between melatonin, sleepiness, and body temperature.*

## Author details

Sheikh Saba Naz[1†], Muhammad Muddassar Shafiq[2] and Mohammed Albreiki[3*†]

1 Department of Microbiology, Jinnah University for Women, Pakistan

2 Punjab Rangers Teaching Hospital, Lahore, Pakistan

3 Center for Biotechnology, Khalifa University of Science and Technology, Abu Dhabi, United Arab Emirates

*Address all correspondence to: m.albreiki1987@gmail.com

† These authors contributed equally.

## References

[1] Lok R et al. Light, alertness, and alerting effects of white light: A literature overview. Journal of Biological Rhythms. 2018;**33**(6):589-601

[2] Valdez P. Focus: Attention science: Circadian rhythms in attention. The Yale Journal of Biology and Medicine. 2019;**92**(1):81

[3] Okechukwu CE. The neurophysiologic basis of the human sleep–wake cycle and the physiopathology of the circadian clock: A narrative review. The Egyptian Journal of Neurology, Psychiatry and Neurosurgery. 2022;**58**(1):1-7

[4] Scammell TE. Overview of sleep: The neurologic processes of the sleep-wake cycle. The Journal of Clinical Psychiatry. 2015;**76**(5):26409

[5] Boivin DB et al. Complex interaction of the sleep-wake cycle and circadian phase modulates mood in healthy subjects. Archives of General Psychiatry. 1997;**54**(2):145-152

[6] Markov D, Goldman M. Neurobiologic mechanisms of sleep and wakefulness. Focus. 2014;**12**(1):9-15

[7] Kishi A et al. NREM sleep stage transitions control ultradian REM sleep rhythm. Sleep. 2011;**34**(10):1423-1432

[8] Monti JM. The role of dorsal raphe nucleus serotonergic and non-serotonergic neurons, and of their receptors, in regulating waking and rapid eye movement (REM) sleep. Sleep Medicine Reviews. 2010;**14**(5):319-327

[9] Saper CB et al. Sleep state switching. Neuron. 2010;**68**(6):1023-1042

[10] Charloux A et al. Aldosterone release during the sleep-wake cycle in humans. American Journal of Physiology-Endocrinology and Metabolism. 1999;**276**(1):E43-E49

[11] Fuller PM, Gooley JJ, Saper CB. Neurobiology of the sleep-wake cycle: Sleep architecture, circadian regulation, and regulatory feedback. Journal of Biological Rhythms. 2006;**21**(6):482-493

[12] Czeisler CA, Gooley JJ. Sleep and circadian rhythms in humans. In: Cold Spring Harbor Symposia on Quantitative Biology. New York, USA: Cold Spring Harbor Laboratory Press; 2007

[13] Carskadon MA. Guidelines for the multiple sleep latency test (MSLT): A standard measure of sleepiness. Sleep. 1986;**9**(4):519-524

[14] Doghramji K et al. A normative study of the maintenance of wakefulness test (MWT). Electroencephalography and Clinical Neurophysiology. 1997;**103**(5):554-562

[15] Johns MW. A new method for measuring daytime sleepiness: The Epworth sleepiness scale. Sleep. 1991;**14**(6):540-545

[16] Shahid A et al. ZOGIM-A (Alertness Questionnaire). In: STOP, THAT and One Hundred Other Sleep Scales. New York, USA: Springer; 2011. pp. 405-406

[17] Shahid A et al. Toronto Hospital Alertness Test (THAT). In: STOP, THAT and One Hundred Other Sleep Scales. New York, USA: Springer; 2011. pp. 391-392

[18] Hoddes E, Zarcone V, Dement W. Stanford sleepiness scale. Enzyklopädie der Schlafmedizin. 1972;**1184**:1

[19] Vitaterna MH, Takahashi JS, Turek FW. Overview of circadian rhythms. Alcohol Research & Health. 2001;**25**(2):85

[20] Cajochen C, Chellappa SL, Schmidt C. Circadian and light effects on human sleepiness–alertness. In: Sleepiness and Human Impact Assessment. Milano, Italy: Springer; 2014. pp. 9-22

[21] Posner M, Rafal R. Neuropsychological Rehabilitation. USA: MJ Meier, A; 1987

[22] Posner MI, Petersen SE. The attention system of the human brain. Annual Review of Neuroscience. 1990;**13**(1):25-42

[23] Schmidt C et al. A time to think: Circadian rhythms in human cognition. Cognitive Neuropsychology. 2007;**24**(7):755-789

[24] McHill AW et al. Chronic sleep curtailment, even without extended (> 16-h) wakefulness, degrades human vigilance performance. Proceedings of the National Academy of Sciences. 2018;**115**(23):6070-6075

[25] Zeeuw JD et al. The alerting effect of the wake maintenance zone during 40 hours of sleep deprivation. Scientific Reports. 2018;**8**(1):1-11

[26] Gallegos C et al. Circadian and homeostatic modulation of the attentional blink. Chronobiology International. 2019;**36**(3):343-352

[27] Smith KJ, Valentino DA, Arruda JE. Measures of variations in performance during a sustained attention task. Journal of Clinical and Experimental Neuropsychology. 2002;**24**(6):828-839

[28] Foster RG. Sleep, circadian rhythms and health. Interface Focus. 2020;**10**(3):20190098

[29] Figueiro MG et al. Light at night and measures of alertness and performance: Implications for shift workers. Biological Research for Nursing. 2016;**18**(1):90-100

[30] Chellappa SL, Gordijn MC, Cajochen C. Can light make us bright? Effects of light on cognition and sleep. Progress in Brain Research. 2011;**190**:119-133

[31] Contreras JD, Eisenberg JN. Does basic sanitation prevent diarrhea? Contextualizing recent intervention trials through a historical lens. International Journal of Environmental Research and Public Health. 2020;**17**(1):230

[32] Albreiki M et al. Acute impact of light at night and exogenous melatonin on subjective appetite and plasma leptin. Frontiers in Nutrition. 2022;**2022**:9

[33] Sunde E et al. Alerting and circadian effects of short-wavelength vs. long-wavelength narrow-bandwidth light during a simulated night shift. Clocks & Sleep. 2020;**2**(4):502-522

[34] Silvani MI, Werder R, Perret C. The influence of blue light on sleep, performance and wellbeing in young adults: A systematic review. Frontiers in Physiology. 2022;**2022**:1485

[35] Prevention CfDCa. The colour of the light affects circadian rhythms 2020 [cited 2022 Dec 22]. 2020. Available from: https://www.cdc.gov/niosh/emres/longhourstraining/color.html

[36] Lin J, Westland S, Cheung V. Effect of intensity of short-wavelength light on electroencephalogram and subjective alertness. Lighting Research & Technology. 2020;**52**(3):413-422

[37] Ahammed GJ et al. Endogenous melatonin deficiency aggravates high temperature-induced oxidative

stress in Solanum lycopersicum L. Environmental and Experimental Botany. 2019;**161**:303-311

[38] Osilla EV, Marsidi JL, Sharma S. Physiology, Temperature Regulation. Florida, USA. 2018

[39] Tan CL, Knight ZA. Regulation of body temperature by the nervous system. Neuron. 2018;**98**(1):31-48

[40] Okamoto M, Mizuno K. Effects of thermal environment on sleep and circadian rhytm. Journal of Physiological Anthropology. 2012;**31**:14

[41] Parmeggiani PL. Interaction between sleep and thermoregulation: An aspect of the control of behavioral states. Sleep. 1986;**10**(5):426-435

[42] Okamoto-Mizuno K et al. Effects of low ambient temperature on heart rate variability during sleep in humans. European Journal of Applied Physiology. 2009;**105**(2):191-197

[43] Vellei M et al. Human thermal perception and time of day: A review. Temperature. 2021;**8**(4):320-341

[44] Harding EC, Franks NP, Wisden W. The temperature dependence of sleep. Frontiers in Neuroscience. 2019;**13**:336

[45] Alföldi P et al. Brain and core temperatures and peripheral vasomotion during sleep and wakefulness at various ambient temperatures in the rat. Pflügers Archiv. 1990;**417**(3):336-341

[46] Szymusiak R, Gvilia I, McGinty D. Hypothalamic control of sleep. Sleep Medicine. 2007;**8**(4):291-301

[47] Eban-Rothschild A et al. VTA dopaminergic neurons regulate ethologically relevant sleep–wake behaviors. Nature Neuroscience. 2016;**19**(10):1356-1366

[48] Goldstein N et al. Hypothalamic neurons that regulate feeding can influence sleep/wake states based on homeostatic need. Current Biology. 2018;**28**(23):3736-3747

[49] Cowley MA et al. Leptin activates anorexigenic POMC neurons through a neural network in the arcuate nucleus. Nature. 2001;**411**(6836):480-484

[50] Everson CA, Bergmann BM, Rechtschaffen A. Sleep deprivation in the rat: III. Total sleep deprivation. Sleep. 1989;**12**(1):13-21

[51] Prete FR et al. Sleep deprivation in the rat: XII. Effect on ambient temperature choice. Sleep. 1991;**14**(2):109-115

[52] Zaki NF et al. Sleep and circadian rhythms in health and disease: A complex interplay. European Archives of Psychiatry and Clinical Neuroscience. 2019;**269**:365-366

[53] Refinetti R. The circadian rhythm of body temperature. Frontiers in Bioscience-Landmark. 2010;**15**(2):564-594

[54] Nam D, Yechoor VK, Ma K. Molecular clock integration of brown adipose tissue formation and function. Adipocytes. 2016;**5**(2):243-250

[55] Coiffard B et al. A tangled threesome: Circadian rhythm, body temperature variations, and the immune system. Biology. 2021;**10**(1):65

[56] Weinert D, Waterhouse J. The circadian rhythm of core temperature: Effects of physical activity and aging. Physiology & Behavior. 2007;**90**(2-3):246-256

[57] Kelly G. Body temperature variability (Part 1): A review of the history of body temperature and its variability due to site selection, biological rhythms, fitness, and aging. Alternative Medicine Review. 2006;**11**(4):278-293

[58] Baker FC et al. Sleep and 24 hour body temperatures: A comparison in young men, naturally cycling women and women taking hormonal contraceptives. The Journal of Physiology. 2001;**530** (Pt 3):565

[59] te Kulve M et al. The influence of light on thermal responses. Acta Physiologica. 2016;**216**(2):163-185

[60] Cajochen C et al. High sensitivity of human melatonin, alertness, thermoregulation, and heart rate to short wavelength light. The Journal of Clinical Endocrinology & Metabolism. 2005;**90**(3):1311-1316

[61] Burgess HJ et al. Effects of bright light and melatonin on sleep propensity, temperature, and cardiac activity at night. Journal of Applied Physiology. 2001;**91**(3):1214-1222

[62] Morita T, Tokura H. Effects of lights of different color temperature on the nocturnal changes in core temperature and melatonin in humans. Applied Human Science. 1996;**15**(5):243-246

[63] Rüger M et al. Nasal versus temporal illumination of the human retina: Effects on core body temperature, melatonin, and circadian phase. Journal of Biological Rhythms. 2005;**20**(1):60-70

[64] Ishibashi K et al. Thermoregulatory effect in humans of suppressed endogenous melatonin by pre-sleep bright-light exposure in a cold environment. Chronobiology International. 2010;**27**(4):782-806

[65] Atkinson G et al. Bright light and thermoregulatory responses to exercise. International Journal of Sports Medicine. 2008;**29**(03):188-193

[66] Kim H-E, Tokura H. Influence of two different light intensities from 16: 00 to 20: 30 hours on evening dressing behavior in the cold. Collegium Antropologicum. 2007;**31**(1):145-151

[67] Aizawa S, Tokura H. Influence of bright light exposure for several hours during the daytime on cutaneous vasodilatation and local sweating induced by an exercise heat load. European Journal of Applied Physiology and Occupational Physiology. 1998;**78**(4):303-307

[68] Seika A, Hiromi T. The influence of bright light exposure for several hours during daytime on tympanic temperature level at sweating onset. Journal of Thermal Biology. 1998;**23**(2):99-106

[69] Marrin K et al. A meta-analytic approach to quantify the dose–response relationship between melatonin and core temperature. European Journal of Applied Physiology. 2013;**113**(9):2323-2329

[70] Cook JS, Sauder CL, Ray CA. Melatonin differentially affects vascular blood flow in humans. American Journal of Physiology-Heart and Circulatory Physiology. 2011;**300**(2):H670-H674

[71] Cagnacci A, Elliott J, Yen S. Melatonin: A major regulator of the circadian rhythm of core temperature in humans. The Journal of Clinical Endocrinology & Metabolism. 1992;**75**(2):447-452

[72] Van Den Heuvel CJ, Kennaway DJ, Dawson D. Thermoregulatory and soporific effects of very low dose

melatonin injection. American Journal of Physiology-Endocrinology and Metabolism. 1999;**276**(2):E249-E254

[73] Satoh K, Mishima K. Hypothermic action of exogenously administered melatonin is dose-dependent in humans. Clinical Neuropharmacology. 2001;**24**(6):334-340

[74] Lockley SW et al. Short-wavelength sensitivity for the direct effects of light on alertness, vigilance, and the waking electroencephalogram in humans. Sleep. 2006;**29**(2):161-168

[75] Figueiro MG et al. Preliminary evidence that both blue and red light can induce alertness at night. BMC Neuroscience. 2009;**10**(1):1-11

[76] Plitnick B et al. The effects of red and blue light on alertness and mood at night. Lighting Research & Technology. 2010;**42**(4):449-458

[77] Cajochen C et al. Thermoregulatory effects of melatonin in relation to sleepiness AU-Kräuchi. Kurt Chronobiological International. 2006;**23**:475-484

[78] Pranil T, Moongngarm A, Loypimai P. Influence of pH, temperature, and light on the stability of melatonin in aqueous solutions and fruit juices. Heliyon. 2020;**6**(3):e03648

[79] Lok R et al. Daytime melatonin and light independently affect human alertness and body temperature. Journal of Pineal Research. 2019;**67**(1):e12583

Chapter 2

# The Relationships of Age-Related Changes in the Biorhythms of the Thymus Endocrine Function and Pineal Melatonin-Producing Function in Healthy People

*Irina Labunets*

## Abstract

The circadian and circannual rhythms play the main role in the adaptation of human immune and pituitary-adrenal systems functioning to the changing photoperiod. The rhythmicity of thymus endocrine function is an important part of the chronobiological organization of immune system. The pineal hormone melatonin is the central regulator of rhythms of healthy human organism functions and involves thymus hormones (namely FTS/thymulin) in synchronizing influence on the immune system functioning. Age-related changes of thymus hormone and melatonin rhythms in healthy people are linked and precede the aging desynchronosis of immune and pituitary-adrenal system functions. In healthy male versus female the above changes occur at earlier life periods and are more pronounced. The thymus endocrine function does not completely disappear in the elderly/old people and is able to respond to the synchronizing influence of melatonin with part of the adrenal gland. Age-related changes in the circadian and circannual rhythms of the thymus hormone, melatonin, immune system, and adrenal gland functions become more pronounced at the development of age-associated diseases (neurodegenerative, cardiovascular, oncological). Melatonin can be perspective medicine for restoration of disturbed rhythmicity of thymus, immune system, and adrenal glands in accelerated human aging and in patients with age-dependent diseases.

**Keywords:** thymus hormones, pineal gland melatonin, human biorhythms, age, age-related diseases

## 1. Introduction

Time-dependent rhythmicity in the organization of physiological processes is an important property of living organisms [1]. Circadian (daily) and circannual (seasonal) rhythms play the main role in human organism adaptation to such changing environmental factors as light, temperature, geomagnetic field, and humidity [1, 2].

Among the above factors, the photoperiod has the most stable synchronizing properties for circadian and circannual rhythms of different human organs and system functions. The circadian rhythms provide fast adaptation of organism functions to the day-night shifts, whereas the circannual rhythms control potential possibilities of functions and differentiation processes.

The control system of these rhythms includes the next components: (a) generator (pacemaker) of endogenous rhythms of functions (suprachiasmatic nucleus (SCN) of the hypothalamus), (b) afferent way to the pacemaker and (c) efferent pathway from the pacemaker to peripheral organs [1, 3]. The pineal gland hormone melatonin plays a key role in the regulation of human circadian and circannual rhythms of organism functions through the coordination of endogenous rhythms that are generated in SCN [4, 5]. In adult organisms melatonin production during the dark period and with the shortening season photoperiod increases.

The circadian and circannual rhythms of immune system indices in healthy young/adult human subjects are found [6–9]. Human immune system functions are under the influence of thymus hormones [10]. The thymus endocrine function is characterized by circadian rhythm and melatonin is responsible for its nocturnal increase [11].

In aging there occurs dyscoordination of rhythms and disturbance of adaptive capacity of the immune and neuroendocrine systems which are associated with the development of age-related diseases [12]. Age-dependent changes in the thymus and pineal gland functioning precede the aging disturbances of the above systems and influence lifespan [4, 10]. At the same time, the administration of melatonin and thymus hormones to aging people leads to a decrease not only in age changes in immune and neuroendocrine system functions but also in the incidence of age-related diseases [13, 14].

This chapter of the monograph reviews the published and our own data about circadian and circannual rhythms of the thymus hormonal function and the pineal melatonin-producing function in young/adult healthy human, their changes in aging, and link with disturbances in rhythmicity of immune and neuroendocrine systems. A connection was shown between age desynchronosis of the thymus and pineal gland functioning, on the one hand, and the development of some age-related diseases, on the other hand. The significance of the maintenance of rhythmicity of immune-neuroendocrine interactions involving thymus and pineal gland in the activation of adaptive features of the human organism is substantiated.

## 2. Thymus as a regulator of immune system functions in healthy human organism

### 2.1 Young/adult people

#### *2.1.1 Cytocrine and endocrine thymus functions*

##### *2.1.1.1 T cells differentiation*

Different subpopulations of T lymphocytes with certain functional properties (T effectors/suppressors, T helpers) are formed in the thymus [15–19]. "Maturation" of T cells in thymus begins from the migration of their progenitors (prothymocytes) from bone marrow. After "maturation" T cell subpopulations (CD4+ and CD8+ T cells) migrate from thymus to T-dependent zones of spleen and lymphoid nodes and bone marrow [18, 19]. Small amounts of immature T cells also migrate from thymus to peripheral lymphoid organs where they can differentiate into mature cells. A more detailed description of thymus cytocrine function is presented in the book review [20].

Along with cytocrine function, the thymus acts as an endocrine organ. It is known that true hormones, including the thymus hormones, must meet the following criteria:

- formation by specialized glandular cells mainly or exclusively in the endocrine gland (for the thymus by epithelial cells);
- secretion into the circulating fluids, determination in the bloodstream, and disappearance from it after gland removal (thymectomy for the thymus);
- specific and high biological activity (biologically active concentration in the circulation);
- the effects mainly outside gland (for thymus—influence on bone marrow, peripheral lymphoid organs, and circulating T-lymphocytes);
- loss of gland function after its removal and recovery after administration of its factors (change in T lymphocyte functions after thymus removal and their restoration by thymus factors).

Only a few of the numerous peptides of the thymus meet the criteria for true hormones. It was shown that the thymus produces the next hormones: thymosin-α1, thymopoetin II, and thymulin/thymic serum factor (FTS) [15, 21–24].

#### *2.1.1.2 Thymosin-α1*

Thymosin-α1 was found in medullary epithelial cells and Hassal's bodies of the human thymus just like in blood [21, 25]. Besides, thymosin-α1 is formed in other lymphoid and non-lymphoid tissues of humans [26]. Hormone blood content decreases after thymus removal and with age [27]. Thymosin-α1 influence on T lymphocytes differentiation in the thymus and the activity of mature peripheral immune cells (antibodies production, change in lymphocytes proliferation) increases interleukin (IL)-10 production and decreases the content of blood tumor necrosis factor α (TNF-α) and IL-6 [21]. Thymosin-α1 due to its immunomodulatory properties is already used in the clinical treatment of infectious diseases, immunodeficiency, and cancer [28].

#### *2.1.1.3 Thymopoietins*

The discovery of thymopoietins was associated with the study of neuromuscular transmission in severe myasthenia gravis and significant therapeutic effect after thymectomy [22]. Along with its influence on neuromuscular transmission, thymopoietins modulate the expression of membrane molecules on immature T cells (induction differentiation of prothymocytes to thymocytes) and enhance manifestations of T-immune defense [22, 29]. Thymopoietins are ubiquitously produced, mainly by immune system organs (including thymus) and are determined in the blood [27]. Its serum content begins to decrease around 10 years of age [27].

So, thymosins and thymopoietins can be attributed to the true thymus hormones, since they are secreted by the epithelial cells of the thymus, are found in the blood, and influence differentiation of T-lymphocytes and their activity. A more detailed description of these hormones' properties is presented in a number of reviews [21, 22, 30].

#### *2.1.1.4 Thymulin/FTS*

Among the thymus hormones, of particular interest is the highly biologically active FTS/thymulin with a $Zn^{2+}$-dependent activity. It is formed exclusively in the thymic epithelial cells of humans and animals, circulates in the blood, disappears from circulation after thymectomy and shows biological properties of all known thymus hormones [23, 31, 32]. FTS influences all stages of differentiation of T lymphocytes (bone marrow, thymus, peripheral lymphoid organs). Thus, in the bone marrow suboptimal doses of FTS act on the expression of CD90 (Thy-1 antigens), CD2, CD5, and CD7 markers on the progenitors of T lymphocytes [15]. Expression of these markers on T cells progenitors characterizes an increase in their ability to migration and adhesion [16]. FTS also acts as a chemotactic signal that plays a role in the migration of bone marrow T-cell progenitors into thymus.

In the thymus FTS affects thymocyte antigen-1 (Thy-1) and cluster of differentiation 3 protein (CD3) expression and influences the balance of regulatory T lymphocytes, cytokine production by CD4+ thymocytes, and transformation of cortisol-sensitive thymocytes into cortisol-resistant ones [15]. Besides, under the FTS influence, there appear markers of mature T lymphocytes on immature cells in the lymph nodes.

FTS affects the functional activity of "mature" T-lymphocytes in peripheral lymphoid organs. Thus, it enhances the proliferative response of T cells to mitogen (phytohemagglutinin) and keeps the regulatory T cells balance, namely helper T cells type 1 and type 2, and increases the number of cytotoxic T cells [33]. FTS enhances the production of interferon γ (IFN-γ) and IL-2 by T helpers type 1 [34]. FTS effects on immune cells can be mediated via high-affinity specific membrane receptors [23, 31]. Besides, FTS stimulates the activity of natural killer cells and the response of peritoneal macrophages to activating effect of IFN-γ [33].

### *2.1.2 Thymus and bone marrow functioning*

Bone marrow is the central organ of the immune and hematopoietic systems. Bone marrow lymphoid and myeloid lineages of hematopoiesis are derived from the common progenitor—hematopoietic stem cells (HSCs) [35, 36]. Progenitor cells of hematopoiesis in bone marrow differentiate into granulocytes, monocytes/macrophages, thrombocytes, and erythrocytes. Bone marrow cells of the microenvironment, namely stromal fibroblasts, macrophages, T helpers, and B cells play an important role in directed differentiation of HSCs [37, 38]. In particular, T lymphocytes (CD4+) of thymus origin can function as regulatory elements of hematopoiesis producing such cytokines as IL-3,4,5,6,13,17 and granulocyte macrophage colony-stimulating factor (GM-CSF) [18, 37]. In human patients with combined immunodeficiency, recovery of impaired differentiation of bone marrow stem cells in the granulocyte-macrophage direction was observed after injections of bioactive thymus factors [24].

As shown, the thymus is involved in the differentiation of multipotent mesenchymal stromal cells (MMSCs) in the bone marrow. These cells differentiate into osteoblasts, adipocytes, chondrocytes and have immunosuppressive action [39]. Reduced proliferative and osteogenic potentials of MSCs after thymus removal coincides with the decreased amount of bone marrow CD4+ T-cells and lack of thymulin in the blood [40]. At the same time, the above properties of bone marrow MSCs were restored after *in vitro* addition of synthetic FTS [40]. The immunosuppressive effect of bone marrow MSCs was enhanced after thymus removal or after a decrease in its endocrine function [40].

So, the thymus functions are important for the normal functioning of the peripheral immune system and the realization of biological properties of bone marrow HSCs and MSCs in adult organisms. Thymus acts on the bone marrow functions through its hormones and T-lymphocytes. Therefore, thymus dysfunction affects immune defense of the organism against damaging factors of different origins and efficiency of cell therapy using these stem cells.

## 2.2 Elderly/old people

### *2.2.1 Cytocrine and endocrine thymus functions*

Age-related processes in the thymus play a crucial role in changes of immune system functioning in aging [41, 42]. Thymus involution depends on the intra- and extrathymus influences. Intrathymus changes include the degenerative alterations of the epithelial thymus cells, decreased proliferation and enhanced apoptosis of the thymocytes, imbalance in the production of intrathymus cytokines (leukemia inhibitory factor, IL-6, IL-7), blockade of the rearrangement of T cell receptor genes and attenuation of the keratinocyte growth factor production, etc. Age-related deterioration of the thymus epithelial cells structure leads to a decrease in its endocrine function. Age-dependent decrease of the blood serum thymulin level is the most pronounced compared to other thymus hormones [23, 27]. Extrathymus factors of thymus involution may be associated with age-related changes in the neuroendocrine system [41].

The pathways of intrathymus differentiation of thymocytes change with age [43]. Diminished expression of CD3 receptors on the thymocyte membrane may result in age-related changes in T cell selection in the thymus [41]. The peripheral T cell functions (proliferation, cytotoxicity, lymphokine production, etc.) in old humans are worsening [41]. There occurs an imbalance not only between helper and suppressor T cells but also between helper T cells type 1 and type 2 [44]. The range of cytokines being synthesized by these cells is altered thereby stimulating humoral immune response. Besides, the functional activity of neutrophils and mononuclear phagocytes is reduced.

### *2.2.2 Bone marrow functioning*

The proliferative and differentiation potential of HSCs and lymphoid progenitor cells in the bone marrow decreases with age [35, 45]. Alterations of the hematopoiesis are explained by the deterioration of the regulatory mechanisms, accumulation of mutations in cell genome, deoxyribonucleic acid damage and oxidative stress. The shift in the hematopoiesis, namely from lymphopoiesis to myelopoiesis affects blood system functioning and leads to the higher frequency of myeloproliferative disorders.

The proliferative capability of stromal elements in the old bone marrow is changed and an imbalance in their differentiation towards active adipocyte generation can be observed [46]. Aging human MMSCs secrete other cytokines and trophic factors displaying a reduced differentiation potential.

#### *2.2.3 Administration of thymus active factors in aging organism*

The positive effect of thymosin-α1 on immune system is most pronounced in immunodeficiency states (aging, cancer, use of immunosuppressants) [21, 28]. In old patients, following injections of thymus factor thymalin (its structure has sequences that are homologous to thymulin) was observed the increase of diminished blood thymulin level and number of peripheral T cells and neutrophil phagocytic activity [14]. There is evidence that the development of osteoporosis may be linked to an imbalance of regulatory T cells in bone marrow and thymus dysfunction [47]. After thymus factor thymalin administration the reduced spongy bone mineral density increased and bone structure improved in old human subjects [14]. In the old human subjects with thymus endocrine hypofunction, thymus factor administration enhances the differentiation of bone marrow stem cells into macrophages and activates liver macrophages [24], which is associated with a decrease in blood content of small circulating immune complexes [14]. As a result of the long-term circulation of these complexes, the vascular walls are damaged promoting the development of vascular diseases.

In summing up, the thymus biologically active factors produce geroprotective effects in elderly people thereby influencing positively age-related changes in immunological indices and bone marrow functioning.

## 3. Biorhythms of thymus and immune system functions and their age-related changes in healthy people

### 3.1 Circadian rhythms

#### *3.1.1 Thymus*

Studies on the circadian rhythm of thymus endocrine function revealed higher nocturnal thymulin/FTS and thymosin-α1 levels in the blood of healthy young human subjects compared to daytime content [11, 21]. According to our data, the thymus endocrine function in young healthy humans (20–29 years old) is characterized by increased blood FTS content at 21.00 and its highest value at 1.00 am [6, 7, 48, 49]. In elderly healthy people (after 60 years), the nocturnal rise FTS level is less compared to young subjects or the hormone rhythm is monotonous [48–50].

#### *3.1.2 Bone marrow*

The human bone marrow hematopoietic and microenvironment cells have a circadian rhythm [51, 52]. Human HSCs taken for transplantation at evening hours (during thymus function activation) have shown better positive effects compared to morning hours [52].

#### *3.1.3 Peripheral immune system*

In healthy young human subjects, the circadian rhythms in the peripheral blood contents of CD4+ and CD8+ T cells, granulocytes, imunoglobulins (Ig), and some cytokines were observed [6, 53, 54]. Age-related changes in circadian rhythms of immune cells show themselves both in their number and functional activity. Thus, in elderly humans, the nocturnal amplitude of the number of blood T cells and its T helper subpopulation is decreased and daily acrophase of neutrophils content is shifted [12, 54]. At the same time, the nocturnal amount of activated T cells and cell production of IL-1, TNF-α, and IFN-γ are increased. So, the response of certain immunological indices to changed light regimens in old organisms can be linked with thymus dysfunction and is not only diminished but also enhanced.

### 3.2 Circannual rhythms

#### *3.2.1 Thymus*

There are no literature data on age-related changes in the thymus endocrine function in healthy people in different seasons of the year. According to our results, the FTS production by thymus in young healthy men and women is characterized by circannual rhythms [6, 55]. We found that the FTS level in healthy humans at age 20–29 years in summer and autumn is higher compared to other seasons (**Table 1**). FTS levels in women higher compared to men (**Table 1**).

In 30–39 old men the FTS blood content in summer decreases and at the age of over 40 its fluctuations become monotonous. In men, after 60 years the highest FTS level is observed in spring. The season changes in FTS level in elderly women mostly look like those in young women although its values decreased in summer and autumn.

So, age-associated changes in the circannual rhythm of FTS level have sex differences. Thus, the first signs of thymus dysfunction are found in men over 30 years old and become more pronounced with age. Age-related changes in thymus hormonal rhythmicity in healthy women are less significant compared to men. It is important that in elderly people the thymus endocrine function does not completely disappear.

#### *3.2.2 Bone marrow*

In the human bone marrow, season-dependent fluctuations of proliferative activity in hematopoietic progenitor and stromal cells have been established [51, 56]. In healthy young individuals, the highest number of colony-forming unit

| Healthy subjects | Spring | Summer | Autumn | Winter |
|---|---|---|---|---|
| Men | 3.8 ± 0.6 | 4.7 ± 0.3* | 5.2 ± 0.3*,** | 3.3 ± 0.3 |
| Women | 5.8 ± 0.3& | 5.6 ± 0.2& | 7.0 ± 0.4**,& | 4.2 ± 0.5 |

**p < 0.05—winter.*
***p < 0.05—autumn.*
*#p < 0.05—summer.*
*&p < 0.05—men (our data [55]).*

**Table 1.**
*FTS level in blood of healthy 20–29-year-old subjects in different seasons, M ± SE.*

granulocyte-macrophage (CFU-GM) was at the end of summer, and the least MSCs possibility for colony formation in the spring and autumn [56]. According to the authors, the annual changes in the number of bone marrow colony-forming unit fibroblasts (CFU-F) should be considered in cell therapy of patients with bone tissue disturbances. After thymus removal in adult organisms, the number of CFU-GM and CFU-F decrease in seasons of their maximum content in bone marrow [57].

#### *3.2.3 Peripheral immune system*

According to the below authors and our data, in healthy young human subjects the amount of blood CD3+, CD4+, and CD8+ T cells; B cells; and content of Ig have maximal values in autumn [6, 53, 54]. In old healthy human subjects, age-related changes of annual fluctuations of immune indices coincide with seasonal desynchronosis of thymus endocrine function and they are characterized by shifting seasonal peaks of the number of blood CD3+, CD4+T cells, and Ig level from autumn to spring [6, 55].

So, age-related immune system response to photoperiod changes is largely associated with age-dependent desynchronosis of thymus functions and can be explained by the disturbance of interactions with the pineal gland which coordinates such reaction [5, 12].

## 4. Role of the pineal gland in the regulation of thymus and immune system biorhythms in healthy people

### 4.1 The pineal gland biorhythms and their changes in aging

The pineal gland and its hormone melatonin is the main regulator of circadian and circannual rhythms not only in mammals but also in the human organism [5, 58]. Production of melatonin during light period is suppressed whereas in the dark hours is increased. Besides, with shortening of the seasonal photoperiod melatonin production is enhanced [59]. Melatonin regulates endogenic rhythms of organisms that are generated in the SCN of the hypothalamus [5, 58]. Melatonin acts on the activity of the hypothalamus-pituitary system and peripheral endocrine glands through its binding with nucleus and membrane receptors which are identified in various brain and endocrine structures. There is a link between pineal gland functioning, organism adaptation, and lifespan [60].

The circadian rhythm of pineal gland function and its changes in aging were found in humans [4, 61]. In the majority of elderly and old human subjects, the nocturnal peak of blood melatonin level is diminished compared to young people [4, 13]. Elderly human subjects with saved pineal gland melatonin-produced function have higher physical and psychomotor activity as well as expressed circadian rhythms of some functions and lifespan [13, 62]. We also observed a nocturnal peak of blood melatonin concentration in young people and its decrease in aging [48, 63, 64]. Age-related decrease of the nocturnal peak of melatonin content in the pineal gland and blood is explained by the diminished activity of the key enzymes of its synthesis (N- acetyltransferase, hydroxyindol-O-methyltransferase), decrease both in the density of β-adrenergic receptors on the pinealocyte membrane and in the capability of postganglionic sympathetic fibers for synthesis and noradrenaline release [4, 61].

The circannual rhythm of blood and pineal gland melatonin content in old humans is characterized by the decrease of the winter peak of hormone level or the shift of its seasonal acrophase to the spring compared to young people [4]. We also found that melatonin level in the blood of young (20–29 years old) healthy men and women was maximal in winter [55]. According to our data, age-related changes in melatonin blood level rhythmicity have sex differences. Thus, in healthy men aged 30-49 years the seasonal peak of blood melatonin content was in summer and in men after 60 years it was in spring. In men, after 30 years melatonin blood level decreases in winter. In elderly women, the spring increases and the winter decrease of blood melatonin was less than in men.

So, the circannual rhythm of melatonin level changes in the blood of healthy men after 30 years. Desynchronosis of this hormone increases with age. Age-related dysfunction of the pineal gland is less pronounced in women compared to men.

### 4.2 Age-related changes of pituitary-adrenal system biorhythms and its link with pineal gland disfunction in healthy people

The rhythmicity of pituitary-adrenal system functioning undergoes changes due to the modulation of the pineal melatonin-producing function [4, 62, 65, 66]. Thus, in young people, the highest blood contents of such adaptive hormones as adrenocorticotrophic hormone (ACTH) and cortisol are observed in the light period of the day compared to evening and night. According to our data, the blood cortisol level in the elderly healthy people does not differ in the morning and evening [48]. At the same time, the altered circadian rhythms of endocrine glands (in particular, adrenal gland) in old human subjects were improved after melatonin injections [4, 48].

The authors found the seasonal fluctuations of cortisol in the blood of healthy people and its age-related changes [4]. We studied annual fluctuations of blood ACTH and cortisol levels in healthy men and women of different ages [55]. We found that in young healthy men and women (20–29 years old), the highest ACTH level was in spring-summer periods of the year and cortisol in autumn. In 30–39 old men, ACTH level increases in winter and such changes in hormone level were also observed in 40–59 old men. In healthy women (30–59 years old) age-related increase in ACTH level is less intensive and forms later compared to men.

In young healthy men (20–39 years old), the blood cortisol level increases in autumn and winter. After 40 cortisol level significantly increases in spring and its annual rhythm becomes monotonous. The seasonal increase of cortisol content in autumn observed in 20–29-year-old healthy women remains unchanged up to the age of 50. The blood cortisol content in spring and summer is lower in women after 40 than in men of the same age.

So, changes in circannual rhythms of blood melatonin and ACTH levels are seen in men as early as the age of 30–39 years. These changes are ahead of age-related activation of the glucocorticoid function of the adrenal cortex and the formation of its seasonal desynchronosis in elderly people. In healthy men changes in the pituitary-adrenal system are more intense compared to women and are formed earlier [55]. Sex differences in age-related changes of the above system functioning can be explained not only by higher blood melatonin levels in women but also by the neuroprotective and neurotrophic effects of estrogens. Melatonin stimulates neurotransmitters exchanged in the hypothalamus and promotes brain sensitivity to peripheral regulatory signals [5].

Thus, the age pineal gland dysfunction is the pathogenetic link of age-related desynchronosis of the pituitary-adrenal system. Gender and age-related changes in the pineal gland and pituitary-adrenal system functions may be explained by certain sex-related differences in the development of some age-associated diseases (cardiovascular diseases, cancer, osteoporosis, diabetes, etc.) as well as in the medicine pharmacodynamics during treatment.

## 4.3 Melatonin, other hormones, and the immune system functions in healthy people

Immune system functioning is in close interaction with the neuroendocrine system [30, 67]. Melatonin effects on the immune system functions include not only direct ways via own receptors in immune cells but also indirect ways via changing endocrine glands functions [67].

### *4.3.1 Thymus*

Thymus is the first target for melatonin [67]. Melatonin is capable to influence directly on the synthesis and secretion of thymus hormones [67, 68]. Melatonin action on the thymus endocrine function can pass through changes in hypothalamus-pituitary-adrenal axis functioning [69, 70]. High concentrations of glucocorticoids suppress thymus endocrine function [70]. The efficiency of thymus hormone administration is increased under the condition of short-term hypocorticism. Fluctuations of the expression and/or sensitivity of glucocorticoid receptors on the thymus epithelial cells are controlled by melatonin [71]. The lymphocytes and epithelial cells of the thymus have receptors for glucocorticoids and androgens [68]. Corticosteroids influence the differentiation of thymus epithelial cells and sex hormones act on the differentiation of thymocytes via FTS synthesis [72, 73]. Besides, glucocorticoids influence the distribution of mature T-lymphocytes in the organism and their accumulation in bone marrow [18].

The authors' data and our own findings have shown that in young human subjects, the nocturnal peaks of blood thymus hormones level (thymulin/FTS, thymosin-α1) and melatonin are similar [6, 11, 48]. We found that in young healthy men aged 20–29 years, the increase of blood melatonin and FTS levels was at 21.0 p.m. with a peak at about 1.0 a.m. (**Figure 1**), whereas the level of cortisol was lowest at 21.0 p.m. and highest at about 5.0 a.m. and 9.0 a.m. [6, 48].

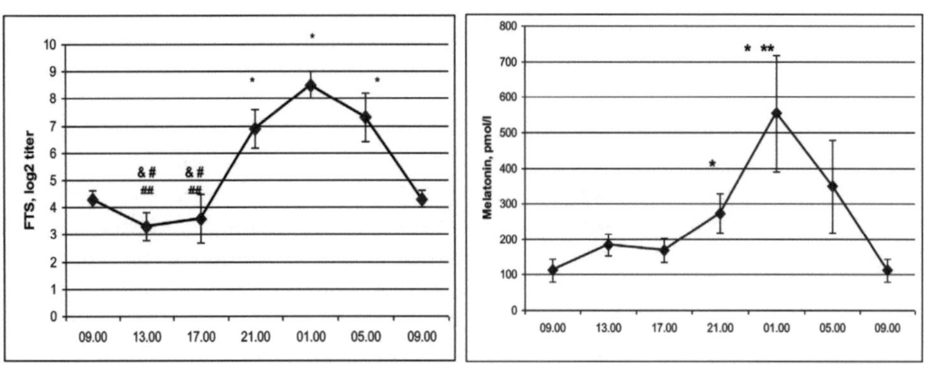


**Figure 1.**
*FTS and melatonin blood levels in healthy young people (aged 20–29 years) during 24 hours (our data [48]).*
*$^{*}p < 0.05$–9.00; $^{**}p < 0.05$–17.00, $^{\#}p < 0.05$–21.00; $^{\#\#}p < 0.05$–1.00; $^{\&}p < 0.05$–5.00.*

In young organisms, pineal gland hypofunction (removal, prolonged lighting) is accompanied by the disappearance of nocturnal peaks of blood thymulin content. On the contrary, melatonin treatment enhances the expression of prothymosin-α1 in the thymus epithelium and restores circadian changes of T cell composition in the thymus after its damage by constant lighting [74].

The daily fluctuations of thymulin and melatonin blood levels coincide and are characterized by increased values in the evening and highest values at 1.00 a.m. In the morning, the content of these hormone decreases compared to the night period.

In aging organisms, following melatonin injections the nocturnal peak of thymulin blood level, the blood zinc and IL-2 contents were increased and the number of thymus apoptotic cells and the glucocorticoid blood levels were decreased [75, 76]. According to our data, in the elderly subjects, the circadian rhythm of blood FTS was ambiguous and correlated with the patterns of melatonin blood rhythmicity [48, 49, 63]. Thus, an increase in FTS level during dark hours (21.0 p.m. or 3.0 a.m.) coincides with a more pronounced nocturnal increase of blood melatonin content compared to elderly people without thymus activation in dark hours. Besides, our own finding of two-week melatonin injections to elderly human healthy subjects demonstrates an increase in FTS levels in the evening and at night and a decrease in blood cortisol and testosterone levels in the evening [48–50]. In the comparison with our younger patients, this effect was registered with lesser melatonin doses [50]. A melatonin-like synchronizing effect on blood FTS and cortisol levels in elderly people was shown by us for pineal gland peptides [77]. The melatonin level after administration of pineal gland peptides (epithalamin, epithalon) increases in the body [14].

#### *4.3.2 Bone marrow*

Melatonin influence on hematopoiesis is realized directly via the receptors in monocytes/macrophages cells and owing to an increased response of these cells to activating hematopoiesis cytokines, namely IL-3, 4, 6 or GM-CSF [74]. Bone marrow T cells progenitors and T helpers type 1 are the main targets for melatonin [67]. Melatonin synthesized by human bone marrow cells protects *in situ* cells against oxidative stress and enhances the functional activity of the lymphocytes [74]. Pineal gland hypofunction is accompanied by diurnal desynchronosis in the bone marrow functioning.

Our studies have established thymus involvement in melatonin influence on circannual changes of the number of MMSC, CFU-GM as well as CD3+, CD4+, and CD8+ T cells in the bone marrow of young and old organisms [78]. In adult organisms, exogenous melatonin acts on bone marrow cells of the microenvironment and this action is realized via thymus hormone. In old organisms, the participant of thymus hormone in action of melatonin is mainly linked with bone marrow CFU-GM changes.

#### *4.3.3 Peripheral immune system*

Under the influence of exogenous melatonin (evening injections) the number of CD3+ and CD4+ T lymphocytes increased and that of CD8+ T cells decreased in the blood and lymphoid organs; balance not only of CD3+ and CD4+ T cells but also of T helpers type 1 and type 2 was changed and the number of mature B cells in the lymphoid organs and functional activity of the macrophages increased [67, 74]. Melatonin also influences circannual rhythms of the immune system. We have shown that in elderly human subjects after melatonin injections FTS blood level, the amount of blood CD3+ and CD4+ cells, and the phagocytic activity of neutrophils are increased in autumn, being similar to those being seen in the younger subjects [48]. Adrenal and sex hormones also influence cellular and humoral immune responses and phagocytosis.

So, the above data show the pathogenic significance of pineal melatonin-producing dysfunction for age-related changes of thymus and immune system rhythmicity and involvement of adrenal glands and gonads in the synchronizing effect of melatonin.

It is important that along with produced hormones, a number of cytokines are formed in the thymus, for example, TNF-α, IL-1,3,6,7,8,15, IFN-γ, and GM-CSF [79]. All types of thymus cells are able to produce cytokines both spontaneously and after stimulation. But the main producers of cytokines in the thymus are epithelial cells and thymocytes [80]. Intrathymic cytokines are important at various stages of activation, proliferation, and differentiation of thymocytes [80].

Some intrathymic cytokines are involved in the interactions between the thymus and pineal gland. Among such intrathymic cytokines, TNF- α is of particular interest. This cytokine has pronounced pro-inflammatory properties and is considered as a key factor in the pineal-immune axis [30]. TNF-α is secreted by cultured mouse thymocytes, indicating its importance for the development and/or regulation of the immune response [81]. The ability of TNF-α to influence melatonin secretion by the pineal gland has been shown in Ref. [82]. Thus inhibitory effects of this cytokine *in vitro* are realized at the level of transcription factors and manifest themselves in a decrease of N-acetylserotonin and N-acetyltransferase synthesis. The disappearance of the inhibitory effect of TNF-α after its prolonged incubation with the pineal gland suggests the involvement of melatonin in the different phases of the inflammatory process.

In addition, there are data on the stimulating effect of IFN-γ and CSF-GM *in vitro* on the secretion of melatonin by the pineal gland [83].

Therefore, the interaction of melatonin and thymus can be realized not only through thymus hormones but also intrathymic cytokines.

### 4.4 Reverse effects of thymus hormones on neuroendocrine system

Regarding the immune-endocrine interactions, the lymphokines and monokines act as afferent signals for the hypothalamus-pituitary-adrenal axis. Besides, thymulin, thymopoetin, thymosin, and thymic humoral factors are believed to link the immune and central nervous systems [69, 84]. Thus, after injections of thymulin and thymosin fraction 5, the blood ACTH and corticosterone levels increase in adult organisms [68]. In conditions of thymus hypofunction, thymulin gene therapy restores the decreased blood follicle-stimulating hormone and luteinizing hormone (LH) levels, whereas thymosin-β4 stimulates the production of LH in the pituitary gland [85, 86]. Thymulin is believed to be the pituitary trophic peptide [86]. Thymus factors can directly change corticosteroid secretion by adrenal glands in organisms of different ages.

We found the reverse influence of the thymus hormone on the pineal functioning in young organisms [87]. The *in vivo* and *in vitro* studies showed that this influence depends on season and age. Thus, the seasonal dependence of blood melatonin level on thymus factor administration is absent in old *versus* adult organisms. The *in vitro* studies show that the activating effect of synthetic FTS on melatonin production by the pineal gland is also absent in old organisms [87]. Age-related decrease in the pineal gland response to thymus hormone can be associated with the development of structural disturbances in the gland [61]. Moreover, the endocrine balance of aging organisms may play a role in the appearance of changes in the seasonal reaction of pineal melatonin-producing function to thymus factor injections. In aging the excess of glucocorticoids diminishes the melatonin-producing function of the pineal gland and the activating influence of thymus factors on this gland.

So, thymus hormones are an important component in immune-neuroendocrine interactions in adult organisms. In aging the reverse effects of thymus hormones on the neuroendocrine system are disturbed.

## 5. Age-related changes in the thymulin/FTS and melatonin biorhythms in human age-associated pathologies

As was shown in previous sections, circadian and circannual rhythms play an important role in the adaptive reactions of human neuroendocrine and immune systems to changing photoperiods. The rhythms of these systems are disturbed in human aging and are linked with altered rhythmicity of melatonin and thymus hormone production. The development of age-dependent diseases may be associated with the intensification or acceleration of age-related changes in the immune and neuroendocrine systems functions.

### 5.1 Neurodegenerative diseases

The frequency of age-related neurodegenerative pathology, such as Parkinson's disease (PD), Alzheimer's disease (AD), brain ischemia, and multiple sclerosis (MS) increases worldwide and has great socio-economic implications. Progressive neurons loss was shown in neurodegenerative diseases. Their development includes enhancement of oxidative stress, neuroinflammation along with microglia activation, mitochondrial dysfunction, disturbances of brain neurogenesis, sleep-wake cycle, and immune system functions. It is important that along with its influence on the neuroendocrine system functions, thymus hormone thymulin has anti-inflammatory effects on the central nervous system, reducing the synthesis of pro-inflammatory cytokines [88].

#### *5.1.1 Alzheimer's disease*

A more pronounced age-related decrease of the nocturnal blood melatonin content in AD elderly patients compared to the control group are coincided with the development of daily desynchronosis of blood ACTH and cortisol levels and cognitive disturbances [66, 89]. Circadian changes in organism functions often occur at early stages of AD and may precede the appearance of cognitive symptoms. Infiltration of active T lymphocytes and mononuclear phagocytes into the injured brain was shown in AD [90]. Melatonin treatment improves disturbed sleep rhythm and produces synchronizing, antioxidant anti-inflammatory and immunomodulatory effects in this pathology [89].

#### *5.1.2 Parkinson's disease*

PD is characterized by circadian disturbances in blood melatonin and cortisol levels compared to the elderly healthy control group as well as the disturbed sleep rhythm [91]. PD development is slowed after melatonin administration which may be linked with its chronobiological, antioxidant and anti-inflammatory effects [92]. Active peripheral T cells, macrophages, and neutrophils infiltrate the brain and damage dopaminergic neurons [93]. In our study, the immune disturbances in parkinsonism were connected with the decrease of blood thymulin level which is restored after melatonin administration [94]. The gender differences in the frequency and clinical symptoms were found in neurodegenerative diseases. Thus, more men than women suffer from PD. These sex differences may be linked with estrogen neurotrophic influence on brain, in particular neurons in SCN. In our data, the women had less intensive and slower age-related development of circannual rhythms disorders in blood FTS, melatonin, ACTH, and cortisol levels compared to men [55].

#### *5.1.3 Brain ischemia*

In the elderly ischemic stroke patients the nocturnal melatonin content is decreased compared to the age control group and is associated with elevated blood cortisol levels and altered sleep-wake rhythm [95]. Peripheral T cells may migrate into the injured brain, release pro-inflammatory cytokines and chemokine and cause further injury to the ischemic brain [96]. In cerebral ischemia, exogenous melatonin reveals antioxidant, anti-apoptotic, and anti-inflammatory properties [95]. In our experimental brain ischemia, the decreasing blood FTS and melatonin levels coincided [97].

#### *5.1.4 Multiple sclerosis*

In MS patients, the decrease in melatonin level at night is associated with circadian rhythm sleep disturbances and daily blood cortisol level rhythmicity [98, 99]. The higher frequency of MS relapses in the spring/summer period against the winter season is linked with a more marked decrease in nocturnal melatonin levels in these seasons [99]. Melatonin treatment improves the life quality of MS patients. Activation of immune cells leads to damage of myelin and neurons in MS. At the same time melatonin decreases the formation of pathogenic T helper 17 and stimulates the formation of protective Tr1 regulatory cells and anti-inflammatory cytokine IL-10 [99]. We have shown that exogenous melatonin has neuroprotective, anti-inflammatory, antioxidant, and immunomodulatory effects in demyelinating pathology [100]. It is important that melatonin activates the thymus endocrine function in adult and old organisms with demyelinating pathology and restores thymulin blood levels in autumn.

### 5.2 Cardiovascular diseases

Cardiovascular diseases (ischemic heart disease (IHD), essential hypertension, and myocardial infarction) are the most common causes of disability and mortality worldwide. Risk factors of these diseases (metabolic and alimentary disturbances, hypodynamia, unhealthy habits, psycho-emotional tensions, and inheritance) occur preferably in elderly humans and coincide with changes in the neuro-endocrine and immune systems functions [14]. Thus, in elderly patients with IHD and essential hypertension, the nocturnal blood melatonin content is lower compared to the healthy control group [13]. The degree of pineal gland dysfunction correlates with disturbances in rhythmicity of cardiovascular system indices.

Clinical data indicate an acceleration of age-related changes in peripheral immune system functioning and their role in the development of cardiovascular diseases [13, 14]. The cytokines, activated leucocytes, circulating immune complexes, and macrophages are able to damage artery walls, alter endothelium and change vessel permeability that, in turn, can cause plaque formation in the damaged areas. Positive effects of biologically active thymus factors on some of the above immunological indices were shown [14]. According to our data, in elderly patients with cardiovascular diseases, the types of FTS circadian rhythms were similar to those recorded in the healthy control group [48, 50, 77]. However, the number of patients with monotonous and inverted FTS blood level rhythms was significantly greater than in the age control group in which the people with reduced nighttime hormone levels predominated. Taking melatonin in the evening led to thymus activation and appearance of daily differences in the FTS blood levels due to its increase in the evening. In these patients, the circadian rhythm of blood cortisol levels also improved. So, melatonin administration in the evening delays the onset of aging changes in the rhythmicity of thymus, immune system, and adrenal glands functioning in elderly patients with IHD. Besides, in cardiovascular pathology melatonin produces antioxidant and anti-inflammatory effects [13].

### 5.3 Oncological diseases

The frequency of tumors increases every 5 years in people after 40 years of age. According to the below authors, circadian rhythms the number of blood lymphocytes and their T-populations are destroyed in tumor organisms and seasonal changes in tumor growth are linked with the seasonal fluctuations of immune system functions [101]. In oncological patients, the nocturnal peak of melatonin blood level is decreased and the circadian rhythm of blood cortisol content is monotonous [102].

We have shown that in oncological patients over 50 years of age, the features of the circadian rhythm of blood FTS and cortisol levels are associated with the character of blood melatonin rhythmicity and point to an increase in their age-related changes [6, 7]. In particular, under conditions of increased melatonin blood level at 21.00 compared to 9.00, the FTS level and the amount of T cells also increased in the evening. When melatonin blood rhythm was inverted, the rhythmicity of FTS blood level and T-lymphocyte content was monotonous. In such patients, the scope of daily changes in blood cortisol content exceeded that observed in patients with activation of pineal gland function in the evening.

In the oncological patients aged 20–40 years, the seasonal peak of blood melatonin level was observed in spring but not in winter as in age-matched controls [6, 7, 103]. The rhythm of blood FTS content becomes monotonous compared to the age control subjects and rhythmicity of the number of blood T-lymphocytes inverted with the highest values in the spring. It is important that the features of rhythmicity of pineal gland and thymus functions in cancer patients till 40 years old are similar to those of healthy older people. These results suggest a possible acceleration of age-related changes in the circannual rhythms of the pineal gland and thymus functioning in oncological patients [104].

The interaction of the thymus and pineal gland may appear during the rhythmical activity of the ovaries (menstrual cycle). The authors showed the link between ovarian dysfunction, on the one hand, and reduced longevity and increased tumor incidence in aging organisms, on the other hand [60]. At the same time, administration of melatonin improves ovarian cyclicity, increases immune system functions, and decreases tumor development. We found that in healthy women under 40, the melatonin blood levels were increased during the follicular and luteal phases of the menstrual cycle and those of FTS during the luteal phase [103]. Unchanged blood levels of melatonin and decreased FTS content in the luteal phase of the cycle were typical for women over 40 [103]. So, the thymus is involved in the ovarian cyclicity regulation by melatonin which can be changed in aging.

Thus, age-related changes in the rhythmicity of immune and neuroendocrine systems functions in patients suffering from neurodegenerative, cardiovascular, and oncological diseases are linked with dysfunction of their central regulators, thymus hormones, and melatonin.

## 6. Conclusion

1. The biorhythms play the main role in the adaptation of the human immune system functioning to the changing environmental factors in particular photoperiod. The circadian (daily) and circannual (season) rhythms of immune system indices (blood T cells, granulocytes and cytokines, bone marrow T cells, hematopoietic and microenvironment cells) are found in healthy young/adult human organisms.

2. Thymus hormones regulate immune system functions in healthy people. The rhythmicity (circadian, circannual) of thymus endocrine function (in particular, thymulin/FTS production) is an important part of the chronobiological organization of the immune system.

3. The pineal hormone melatonin is the central regulator of rhythms of healthy human organism functions and involves thymus hormone (namely thymulin) in synchronizing influence on the immune system functioning. Besides, melatonin effects on the thymus and peripheral immune system rhythmicity include not only direct ways via own receptors in immune cells but also indirect ways via changing endocrine glands functions (pituitary-adrenal system). In thymus-pineal gland interactions, the reverse influence of thymus hormone on the rhythm of melatonin production was found.

4. Age-related changes in the circadian and circannual rhythms of immune system functions (peripheral immune system, bone marrow) in healthy people are linked with age-dependent desynchronosis of thymus endocrine function. Age-dependent changes in the rhythm of blood thymulin level have sex differences. Thus, the first signs of thymus dysfunction are found in men over 30 years and become more pronounced with age. Age-related changes in thymus hormonal rhythmicity in healthy women are less significant compared to men. It is important that in elderly/old people the thymus endocrine function does not completely disappear.

5. Melatonin production decreases in healthy people in aging and is coincided with desynchronosis in thymus, bone marrow, and peripheral immune system functioning. Age changes in rhythmicity of pineal gland and thymus endocrine functions are interrelated and precede aging desynchronosis of immune and pituitary-adrenal system functioning. In healthy males versus females the above changes occur at earlier life periods and are more pronounced. The synchronizing

effect of melatonin on thymus hormones is also manifested in elderly/old people, but the reverse effects of thymus hormones on the neuroendocrine system are disturbed.

6. Age-related changes in the circadian and circannual rhythms of the thymus hormone, melatonin, immune system, and pituitary-adrenal system functions become more pronounced at the development of age-associated diseases (neurodegenerative, cardiovascular, oncological). Age-related changes in rhythmicity of immune and neuroendocrine system function in patients suffering from the above diseases are linked with dysfunction of their central regulators, thymus hormones, and melatonin. Besides, the development of age-dependent diseases may be associated with the intensification or acceleration of age-related changes in rhythms of the immune and neuroendocrine systems functions in adverse conditions (in particular, night shift work, permanent lighting, insomnia).

7. New chronobiological approaches to the prevention and treatment of age-dependent diseases (neurodegenerative, cardiovascular, oncological) may be linked with restoration of the aging disturbances in rhythmicity of immune-neuroendocrine interactions involving the thymus and pineal gland. Melatonin can be useful in the treatment of risk groups with accelerated human aging and in patients with age-dependent diseases to restore circadian and circannual rhythms of thymus hormone (thymulin/FTS) production. Besides, exogenous melatonin has neuroprotective, anti-inflammatory, antioxidant effects, and normalizes fat metabolism in pathological conditions.

In conclusion, we hope that this review has shown pathogenic significance of pineal melatonin-producing dysfunction for age-related changes in the thymus and immune and endocrine systems rhythms and pointed to the importance of supporting immune-neuroendocrine interactions rhythmicity in aging and pathology development.

## Acknowledgements

The author thanks her colleague Turta Maya for her assistance in the preparation of an English version of the given review article.

## Conflict of interest

The authors declare no conflict of interest

## Author details

Irina Labunets[1,2]

1 Experimental Modeling Laboratory, Cell and Tissue Technologies Department, Institute of Genetic and Regenerative Medicine, National Scientific Center "M.D. Strazhesko Institute of Cardiology, Clinical and Regenerative Medicine of the National Academy of Medical Sciences of Ukraine", Kyiv, Ukraine

2 Laboratory of Pathophysiology and Immunology, D. F. Chebotarev State Institute of Gerontology of the National Academy of Medical Sciences of Ukraine, Kyiv, Ukraine

*Address all correspondence to: irina_labunets@ukr.net

## References

[1] Reinberg A, Ashkenazi I. Concepts in human biological rhythms. Dialogues in Clinical Neuroscience. 2003;**5**(4):327-342. DOI: 10.31887/DCNS.2003.5.4/areinberg

[2] Duffy JF, Wright KP. Entrainment of the human circadian system by light. Journal of Biological Rhythms. 2005;**20**(4):326-338. DOI: 10.1177/0748730405277983

[3] Erren TC, Reiter RJ. Defining chronodisruption. Journal of Pineal Research. 2009;**46**(3):245-247. DOI: 10.1111/j.1600-079X.2009.00665.x

[4] Touitou Y. Human aging and melatonin. Clinical relevance. Experimental Gerontology. 2001;**36**(7):1083-1100. DOI: 10.1016/s0531-5565(01)00120-6

[5] Reiter RJ, Rosales-Corral S, Coto-Montes A, Boga JA, Tan DX, Davis JM, et al. The photoperiod, circadian regulation and chronodisruption: Requisite interplay between the suprachiasmatic nuclei and the pineal and gut melatonin. Journal of Physiology and Pharmacology. 2011;**62**(3):269-274

[6] Labunets IF, Grinevich YA. Biological rhythms of immune system functions and possibilities of their regulation in patients with malignant tumours (review of published and authors' own research data). Clinical Oncology. 2014;**2**(14): 46-52. Available from: https://www.clinicaloncology.com.ua/archive

[7] Labunets IF. Changes in melatonin biorhythms and immune-neuroendocrine interactions in oncological patients of different ages. Gerontology & Geriatrics Studies. 2018;**3**(2):GGS.000557.2018. DOI: 10.31031/GGS.2018.03.00057

[8] Scheirmann C, Kunisaki Y, Frenette PS. Circadian control of the immune system. Nature Reviews Immunology. 2013;**13**(3):190-198. DOI: 1038/nri3386

[9] Geiger SS, Fagundes CT, Siegel RM. Chrono-immunology: Progress and challenges in understanding links between the circadian and immune systems. Immunology. 2015;**146**(3):349-358. DOI: 10.1111/imm.12525. Epub: 2015 Sep 28

[10] Csaba G. The immunoendocrine thymus as a pacemaker of lifespan. Acta Microbiologica et Immunologica Hungarica. 2016;**63**(2):139-158. DOI: 10.1556/030.63.2016.2.1

[11] Molinero P, Soutto M, Benot S, Hmadcha A, Guerrero JM. Melatonin is responsible for nocturnal increase observed in serum and thymus of thymosin alpha1 and thymulin concentrations: Observations in rats and humans. Journal of Neuroimmunology. 2000;**103**(2):180-188. DOI: 10.1016/s0165-5728(99)00237-4

[12] Mate I, Madrid JA, De la Fuerite M. Chronobiology of the neuroimmunoendocrine system and aging. Current Pharmaceutical Design. 2014;**20**(29):4642-4655

[13] Korkushko OV, Khavinson VK, Shatilo VB. Handbook of Pineal Gland: Ways for Correction in Aging. St. Petersburg: Nauka; 2006. 204 p. ISBN 5-02-026268-4

[14] Korkushko OV, Khavinson VK, Butenko GM, Shatilo VB. Handbook

of Peptide Preparations of Thymus and Pineal Gland in Prevention of Accelerated Aging. St.-Petersburg: Nauka; 2002. 202 p. ISBN 5-02-026176-9

[15] Yarilin AA, Pinchuk VG, Grinevich YA. Handbook of Structure of Thymus and Differentiation of T Lymphocytes. Kiev: Naukova Dumka; 1991. 248 p. ISBN 5-12-001942-0

[16] Boehm T, Bleul CC. Thymus-homing precursors and the thymic microenvironment. Trends Immunology. 2006;**27**(10):477-484. DOI: 10,1016/j.it.2006.08.004

[17] Alves NL, Huntingto ND, Rodewald HR, Di Santo JP. Thymic epithelial cells: The multitasking framework of the T cell "cradle". Trends Immunology. 2009;**30**(10):468-471. DOI: 10.1016/j.it.2009.07.010

[18] Di Rosa F. T-lymphocyte interaction with stromal, bone and hematopoietic cells in the bone marrow. Immunology and Cell Biology. Cell Biol. 2009;**87**(1):20-29. DOI: 10.1038/icb.2008.84 Epub2008Nov25

[19] Zou L, Barnett B, Safah H, Larussa VF, Evdemon-Hogan M, Mottram P, et al. Bone marrow is a reservoir for CD4+CD25+ regulatory T cell that traffic through CXCL12/CXCR4 signals. Cancer Research. 2004;**64**:8451-8455. DOI: 10.1158/0008-5472.CAN-04-1987

[20] Rezali N, editor. Handbook of Thymus. London; IntechOpen, 2020.144 p. DOI: 10,5772/intechopen.73777

[21] Goldstein AL, Badamchian M. Thymosins: Chemistry and biological properties in health and disease. Expert Opinion in Biological Therapy. 2004;**4**(4):559-573. DOI: 10.1517/14712598.4.4.559

[22] Hadden JW. Thymic endocrinology. Annals of The New York Academy Sciences. 1998;**840**:352-358. DOI: 10.1111/j.1749-6632.1998.tb09574.x

[23] Bach JF, Dardenne M. Studies on thymus products. II. Demonstration and characterization of a circulating thymic hormone Immunology. 1973 Sep;**25**(3):353-366

[24] Trainin N, Pecht M, Handzel ZT. Thymic hormones – inducers and regulators of the T-cell system. Immunology Today. 1983;**4**(1):16-21. DOI: 10.1016/0167-5699(83)90097-X

[25] McClure JE, Lameris N, Wara DW, Goldstein AL. Immunochemical studies on thymosin: Radioimmunoassay of thymosin alpha 1. The Journal of Immunology. 1982;**128**:368-375

[26] Chen C, Li M, Yang H, Chai H, Fisher W, Yao Q. Roles of thymosins in cancers and other organ systems. World Journal of Surgery. 2005;**29**(3):204-270. DOI: 10.1007/s00268-004-7817-2

[27] Bodey B, Bodey B Jr, Siegel SE, Kaiser HE. Involution of the mammalian thymus, one of the leading regulatory of aging. In vivo. 1997;**11**(5):421-440

[28] King R, Tuthill C. Immune modulation with thymosin alpha1 treatment. Vitamins and Hormones. 2016;**102**:151-178. DOI: 10.1016/bs.vh.2016.04.003

[29] Harris CA, Andryuk PJ, Cline S, Chan HK, Natarajan A, Siekierka JJ, et al. Three distinct human thymopoietins are derived from alternatively spliced mRNAs. Proceedings of the National Academy of Sciences of the United States of America. 1994;**91**:6283-6287. DOI: 10.1073/pnas.91.14.6283

[30] Rezzani R, Franco C, Hardeland R, Fabrio LF. Thymus-pineal

gland axis: Revisiting its role in human life and ageing. International Journal of Molecular Sciences. 2020;**21**:806. DOI: 10.3390/ijms21228806

[31] Bach JF, Dardenne M. Thymulin, a zinc-dependent hormone. Medical Oncology and Tumor Pharmacotherapy. 1989;**6**:25-29. DOI: 10.1007/BF02985220

[32] Reggiani PC, Schwerdt JI, Console GM, Roggero EA, Dardenne N, Goya RG. Physiology and therapeutic potential of the thymic peptide thymulin. Current Pharmaceutical Design. 2014;**20**:4690-4696. DOI: 10.2174/1381612820 666140130211157

[33] Prasad AS. Effects of zinc deficiency on Th1 and Th2 cytokine shifts. The Journal of Infectious Diseases. 2000;**182**(Suppl 1):62-68. DOI: 10.1086/315916

[34] Haddad JJ, Saade NE, Safieh-Garabedian B. Thymulin: An emerging anti-inflammatory molecule. Current Medicinal Chemistry. 2005;**4**(3):333-338. DOI: 10.2174/1568014054065195

[35] Geiger H, Rudolf KL. Aging in the lympho-hematopoietic stem cell compartment. Trends Immunology. 2009;**30**(7):360-365. DOI: 10.1016/j.it.2009.03.010

[36] Klein F, Feldhahn N, Lee S, Wang H, Ciuffi F, von Elstermann M, et al. T lymphoid differentiation in human bone marrow. Proceedings of the National Academy of Sciences of the United States of America. 2003;**100**(11):6747-6752. DOI: 10.1073/pnas.1031503100

[37] Monteiro JP, Benjamin A, Costa ES, Barcinski MA, Bonomo A. Normal hematopoiesis is maintained by activated bone marrow CD4+ T cells. Blood. 2005;**105**(4):1484-1491. DOI: 10.1182/blood-2004-07-2856

[38] Ogawa T, Kitagawa M, Hirokawa K. Age-related changes of human bone marrow: A histometric estimation of proliferative cells, apoptotic cells, T cells, B cells and macrophages. Mechanism of Ageing and Development. 2000;**117**:57-68. DOI: 10.1016/s0047-6374(00)00137-8

[39] Li X, Bal J, Ji X, Li R, Xuan Y, Wang Y. Comprehensive characterization of four different populations of human mesenchymal stem cells as regards their immunoproperties, proliferation and differentiation. International Journal of Molecular Medicine. 2014;**34**(3):695-704. DOI: 10.3892/ijmm.2014.1821

[40] Labunets IF, Rodnichenko AE. The effects of different doses thymulin in vivo and in vitro on some biological properties of bone marrow-derived multipotent mesenchymal stromal cells in mice of different strains. Cell and Organ Transplantology. 2018;**6**(1):68-73. DOI: 10.22494/cot.v6i1.82

[41] Hirokawa K, Utsuyama M, Makinodan T. Immunity and aging. In: Pathy MS, editor. Principles and Practice of Geriatric Medicine. 4nd ed. Vol. Vol. 2. New York: J. - Wiley; 2006. pp. 19-36. DOI: 10.1002/9780470090572.ch3

[42] Lynch HE, Goldberg GL, Chidgey A, Van den Brink MR, Boyd R, Sempowski GD. Thymic involution and immune reconstitution. Trends Immunology. 2009;**30**(7):366-373. DOI: 10.1016/j.it.2009.04.003

[43] Thoman LM. The pattern of T lymphocyte differentiation is altered during thymic involution. Mechanism of Ageing and Development. 1995;**82**(2-3):155-170. DOI: 10.1016/0047-6374(95)01597-S

[44] Kidd P. Th1/Th2 balance: The hypothesis, its limitations and implications for health and disease. Alternative Medicine Review. 2003;**8**(3):223-246

[45] Gross L. Mechanisms of aging in bone marrow stem cells. PLoS Biology. 2007;**5**(8):215-216. DOI: 10.1371/journal.pbio.0050215

[46] Fehrer C, Lepperdinger G. Mesenchymal stem cell aging. Experimental Gerontology. 2005;**40**(12):926-930. DOI: 10.1016/j.exger.2005.07.006

[47] Zhao R. Immune regulation of osteoclast function in postmenopausal osteoporosis: A critical interdisciplinary perspective. International Journal of Medical Sciences. 2012;**9**:825-832. DOI: 10.7150/ijms.5180

[48] Labunets IF. Influence of melatonin on biorhythms of functional status of thymus, immune system and adrenal glands cortex in elderly people. Probl Stareniya i Dolgoletiya. 2005;**14**(4):313-322. ISSN 0869-1703. Available from:. http://geront.kiev.ua/psid

[49] Labunets IF. Age-related circadian disturbances in melatonin causing changes in thymus hormones and glucocorticoids rhythmicity in healthy animals and humans. International Journal of Aging Research. 2018;**1**:25. Available from: http://escipub.com/international-journal-of-aging-research/

[50] Antoniuk-Shcheglova IA, Labunets IF, Shatylo VB. Correction of disorders of endocrine function of the thymus by melatonin in the apparently healthy elderly people. Probl Stareniya i Dolgoletiya. 2010;**19**(4):382-387. ISSN 0869-1703. Available from: http://geront.kiev.ua/psid

[51] Smaaland R, Sothern RB, Laerum OD, Abrahamsen JF. Rhythms in human bone marrow and blood cells. Chronobiology International. 2002;**19**(1):101-127. DOI: 10.1081/cbi-120002594

[52] Lucas D, Battista M, Shi PA, Isola L, Frenette PC. Mobilized hematopoietic stem cell yield depends on species-specific circadian timing. Blood. 2008;**112**(11):3494. DOI: 10.1182/blood.v.112.11.3494.3494

[53] Suzuki S, Toyabe S, Moroda T, Tada T, Tsukahara A, Iiai T, et al. Circadian rhythm of leucocytes and lymphocyte subsets and its possible correlation with the function of the autonomic nervous system. Clinical and Experimental Immunology. 1997;**110**:500-508

[54] Born J, Uthgenannt D, Dodt C, Nünninghoff D, Ringvolt E, Wagner T, et al. Cytokine production and lymphocyte subpopulations in aged humans. An assessment during nocturnal sleep. Mechanism of Ageing and Development. 1995;**84**(2):113-126. DOI: 10.1016/0047-6374(95)016384

[55] Labunets IF. Sex peculiarities of age-related changes in circannual rhythms of pineal gland, hypothalamo-pituitary-adrenal axis and thymus in healthy subjects. Advances in Gerontology. 2013;**3**(4):290-296. DOI: 10.1134/s207905701304005X

[56] Astakhova VS, Panchenko LM. Using of cloning methods for discovering the influence of endogermetics action on stroma cells (in vitro). Annals of Mechnicov Institute. 2006;**4**:38-44. ISSN 1993-4327 (online). Available from:. http://nbuv.gov.ua/UJRN/ami_2006_4_9

[57] Labunets IF, Rodnichenko AE, Magdich LV, Butenko GM. The thymus and adaptive changes in the cellular

composition of bone marrow in animals of different ages. Advances in Gerontology. 2012;**2**(1):27-34. DOI: 10.1134/s2079057012010079

[58] Arendt J. Melatonin: Characteristics, concerns, and prospects. Journal of Biological Rhythms. 2005;**20**:291-303. DOI: 10.1177/0748730405277492

[59] Lincoln GA. Melatonin entrainment of circannual rhythms. Chronobiology International. 2006;**23**(1-2):301-306. DOI: 10.1080/07420520500464452

[60] Anisimov VN. Pineal gland, biorhythms and aging of an organism. Uspekhi Fiziologicheskikh Nauk. 2008;**39**(4):40-64

[61] Reiter RJ. Pineal function during aging: Attenuation of the melatonin rhythm and its neurobiological consequences. Acta Neurobiological Experimentalis. 1994;**54**(Suppl):31-39

[62] Ferrari E, Cravello L, Falvo F, Barili L, Solerte SB, Fioravanti M, et al. Neuroendocrine features in extreme longevity. Experimental Gerontolology. 2008;**43**(2):88-94. DOI: 10.1016/j.exger.2007.06.010

[63] Labunets IF. Age-related changes in the melatonin and thymulin biorhythms as risk factors for human neurodegenerative diseases. Gerontollogy & Geriatrics Studies. 2017;**1**(2). DOI: 10.31031/GGS.2017.01.000506

[64] Korkushko OV, Khavinson VK, Shatilo VB, Magdich LV, Labunets IF. Circadian rhythms of pineal gland melatonin forming function in healthy elderly people. Advances in gerontology=Uspekhi gerontologii. 2004;**15**:70-75

[65] Hermann M, Berger P. Hormonal changes in aging men: A therapeutic indication. Experimental Gerontology. 2001;**36**(7):1075-1082. DOI: 10.1016/s0531-5565(00)00160

[66] Ferrari E, Arcaini A, Gornati R, Pelanconi L, Cravello L, Fioravanti M, et al. Pineal and pituitary-adrenocortical function in physiological aging and in senile dementia. Experimental Gerontology. 2000;**35**(9-10):1239-1250. DOI: 10.1016/s05531-5565(00)00160-1

[67] Cardinali DP, Esquifino AJ, Srinivasan V, Pandi-Perumal SR. Melatonin and the immune system in aging. Neuroimmunomodulation. 2008;**15**(4-6):272-278. DOI: 10.1159/000156470

[68] Savino W, Dardenne M. Neuroendocrine control of thymus physiology. Endocrine Reviews. 2000;**21**(4):412-443. DOI: 10.1210/edrv.21.4.0402

[69] Reggiani C, Morel GR, Console GM, Barbeito CG, Rodriguez SS, Brown OA. Thymus–neuroendocrine axis. Physiology, molecular biology, and therapeutic potential of the thymic peptide thymulin. Annals of the New York Academy of Sciences. 2009;**1153**(1):98-106

[70] Savino W, Mendes-da-Cruz DA, Lepletier A, Dardenne M. Hormonal control of T-cell development in health and disease. Nature Reviews Endocrinology. 2016;**12**(2):77-89. DOI: 10.1038/nrendo.2015.168

[71] Saintz RM, Mayo JC, Reiter RJ, Antolin I, Esteban MM, Rodriguez C. Melatonin regulates glucocorticoid receptor: An answer to its antiapoptotic action in thymus. FASEB Journal. 1999;**13**(12):1547-1556. DOI: 10.1096/fasebj.13.12.1547

[72] Hale LP, Markert ML. Corticosteroids regulate epithelial cells differentiation

and hasal body formation in the human thymus. The Journal of Immunology. 2004;**172**:617-624. DOI: 10.4049/jimmunol.172.1.617

[73] Seiki K, Sakabe K. Sex hormones and the thymus in relation to thymocyte proliferation and maturation. Archives of Histology and Cytology. 1997;**60**(1):29-38. DOI: 10.1679/aohc.60.29

[74] Maestroni GJ. The immunotherapeutic potential of melatonin. Expert Opinion Investigational Drugs. 2001;**10**(3):467-476. DOI: 10.1517/13543784.10.3.467

[75] Mocchegiani E, Santarelli L, Tibaldi A, Muzzioli M, Bulian D, Cipriano K, et al. Presence of links between zinc and melatonin during the circadian cycle in old mice: Effects on thymic endocrine activity and on the survival. Journal of Neuroimmunology. 1998;**86**(2):111-122. DOI: 10.1016/s0165-5728(97)00253-1

[76] Tian YM, Zhang GY, Dai YR. Melatonin rejuvenates degenerated thymus and redresses peripheral immune functions in aged mice. Immunology Letters. 2003;**88**(2):101-104. DOI: 10.1016/S0165-2478(03)00068-3

[77] Labunets IF, Butenko GM, Magdich LV, Korkushko OV, Khavinson VK, Shatilo VB. Effect of epithalamin on circadian relationship between the endocrine function of the thymus and melatonin-producing function of the pineal gland in elderly people. Bulletin of Experimental Biology and Medicine. 2004;**137**(5):507-509. DOI: 10.1023/b:bebm.0000038165.09563.b5

[78] Labunets IF, Rodnichenko AE, Butenko GM. Influence of the pineal gland's factors on the cell composition of the bone marrow in animals of different ages in conditions of changed thymus functional state. Advances in Gerontolology= Uspekhi gerontologii. 2011;**24**(1):54-60

[79] Yarilin AA, Belyakov JM. Cytokines in the thymus: Production and biological effects. Current Medicinal Chemistry. 2004;**11**(4):447-464. DOI: 10.2174/0929867043455972

[80] Bodey B, Bodey B Jr, Siegel SE, Kaiser HE. The role of the reticulo-epithelial (RE) cell network in the immuno-neuroendocrine regulation of intrathymic lymphopoiesis. Anticancer Research. 2000;**20**(3A):1871-1888

[81] Giroir BP, Brown T, Beutler B. Consitutive synthesis of tumor necrosis factor in the thymus. The Proceedings of the National Academy of Sciences (PNAS). 1992;**89**(11):4864-4868

[82] Fernandes PACM, Cecon E, Markus RP, Ferreira ZS. Effect of TNF-alpha on the melatonin synthetic pathway in the rat pineal gland: Basis for 'feedback' of the immune response on circadian time. Journal of Pineal Research. 2006;**41**(4):344-350. DOI: 10.1111/j.1600-079X2006.00373.x

[83] Withyachumnarnkul B, Nonaka KO, Santana C, Attia AM, Reiter RJ. Interferon-gamma production in rat modulates melatonin pineal glands in organ culture. Journal of Interferon Research. 1990;**10**(4):403-411. DOI: 10.1089/jir.1990.10.403

[84] Hall NR, McGillis JP, Spangelo BL, Goldstein AL. Evidence that thymosin and other biologic response modifiers can function as neuroactive immunotransmitters. The Journal of Immunology. 1985;**135**:806-811

[85] Goya RG, Reggiani PC, Vesenbeckh SM, Pléau JM, Sosa YE,

Cónsole GM, et al. Thymulin gene therapy prevents the reduction in circulating gonadotropins induced by thymulin deficiency in mice. American Journal of Physiology Endocrinology and Metabolism. 2007;**293**(1):E182-E187. DOI: 10.1152/ajpendo.00085.2007

[86] Goya RJ, Brown OA, Pleau JM, Dardenne M. Thymulin and the neuroendocrine system. Peptides. 2004;**25**(1):139-142. DOI: 10.1016/j.peptides.2003.11.002

[87] Labunets IF. Thymic factors influence on melatonin-producing pineal function in mice of different age: The possible mechanisms. Advances in gerontology=Uspekhi gerontologii. 2007;**20**(1):86-91

[88] Haddad JJ, Hanbali LH. The anti-inflammatory and immunomodulatory activity of thymulin peptide is NF-kB dependent and involves the downregulation of I kB-α. American Journal of Medical and Biological Research. 2013;**1**(2):41-49. DOI: 10.12691/ajmbr-1-2-2

[89] Hardeland R. Melatonin in aging and disease-multiple consequences of reduced secretion, options and limits of treatment. Aging and Disease. 2012;**3**(2):194-225

[90] Town T. Inflammation, immunity and Alzheimer's disease. CNS & Neurological Disorders—Drug Targets. 2010;**9**(2):129-131. DOI: 10.2174/187152710791012008

[91] Lin L, Du Y, Yuan S, Shen J, Lin X, Zheng Z. Serum melatonin is an alternative index of Parkinson's disease severity. Brain Research. 2014;**1547**:43-48. DOI: 10.1016/j.brainres.2013.12.021. Epub 2013 Dec 30

[92] Srinivasan V. Therapeutic potential of melatonin and its analogs in Parkinson's disease: Focus on sleep and neuroprotection. Therapeutic Advances in Neurological Disorders. 2011;**4**(5):297-317. DOI: 10.1177/1756285611406166

[93] Maguire-Zeiss KA, Federoff HJ. Future directions for immune modulation in neurodegenerative disorders: Focus on Parkinson's disease. Journal of Neural Transmission. 2010;**117**(8):1019-1025. DOI: 10.1007/s00702-010-0431-6

[94] Labunets IF. Neuroprotective effects of the pineal hormone melatonin in animals with experimental model of neurodegenerative pathology. In: Handbook of Conceptual Options for the Development of Medical Science and Education: Collective monograph. Riga: Izdevnieciba "Baltija Bublishing"; 2020. pp. 355-370. DOI: 10.30525/978-9934-588-44-0/18

[95] Andrabi SS, Parvez S, Tabassum H. Melatonin and ischemic stroke: Mechanistic roles and action. Advances in Pharmacological Sciences. 2015:384750. DOI: 10.1155/2015/384750

[96] Chengrui A, Yejie S, Peiying L, Xiaoming H, Yu G, Steler RA. Molecular dialogs between the ischemic brain and the peripheral immune system: Dualistic roles in injury and repair. Progress in Neurobiology. 2014;**115**:6-24. DOI: 10.1016/j.pneurobio.2013.12002

[97] Labunets I. Immune-neuroendocrine interactions involving thymus and pineal gland in stem cell therapy of age-related diseases. Immunology, Endocrine & Metabolic Agents in Medicinal Chemistry (IEMAMC). 2015;**15**(2):101-120. DOI: 10.2174/187152221 5666150831203443

[98] Damasceno A, Moraes AS, Farias A, Damasceno BP, dos Santos LM, Cendes F. Disruption of melatonin

circadian rhythm production is related to multiple sclerosis severity: A preliminary study. Journal of the Neurological Sciences. 2015;**353**(1-2):166-168. DOI: 10.1016/j.jns.2015.03.040

[99] Wurtman R. Multiple sclerosis, melatonin and neurobehavioral diseases. Frontiers in Endocrinology. 2017. DOI: 10.3389/fendo.2017.00280

[100] Labunets IF, Rodnichenko AE. Melatonin effects in young and aging mice with the toxic cuprizone-induced demyelination. Advances in Gerontology. 2020;**10**(1):41-49. DOI: 10.1134/S2079057020010105

[101] Nelson RJ, Blom JMC. Photoperiodic effects on tumor development and immune function. Journal of Biological Rhythms. 1994;**9**(3-4):233-249. DOI: 10.1177/074873049400900305

[102] Bartsch C, Bartsch H, Peschke E. Light, melatonin and cancer: Current results and future perspectives. Biological Rhythm Research. 2009;**40**(1):17-35. DOI: 10.1080/09291010802066983

[103] Labunets IF. Age-related biorhythmical disfunction of the pineal gland, thymus and hypophysial-adrenal system in healthy subjects. Aging: Immunology and Infectious Disease. 1996;**6**(3&4):167-176. ISSN: 08928762

[104] Grinevich YA, Labunets IF. Melatonin, thymic serum factor, and cortisol levels in healthy subjects of different age and patients with skin melanoma. Journal of Pineal Research. 1986;**3**(3):263-275. DOI: 10.1111/j.1600-079x.1986.tb00749.x

Chapter 3

# The Progressive Connection among Stress, Anxiety, Sleep, and Neurological Disorders

*Jorge Garza-Ulloa*


## Abstract

Many conditions that can cause "sleep disturbance" for many different health conditions, where normal constant sleep is interrupted since altering falling asleep to a frequent disturbance for a long time duration, usually implicit for a wide range of causes including environment alteration, health problems that affect physical or mental body functions, and others. Finding causes for "*sleep disturbances or sleep disorders*" is not an easy task, even for medical professionals. At this time, where humanity is confronting a huge amount of disasters due to climate change, bacteria and viruses of different kinds have been evolving as a treat with a long pandemic time, and economic impacts do not present a near sign of stabilization; technological advances based on artificial intelligence are making frequent changes in our way of living, which usually widen the amount of information that we receive and process. These factors and others are misdirecting the basic survival needs of human beings, such as food, water, air quality, and the necessary and confronting need to sleep. These altered facts overuse our brains and, as a consequence, maximize their normal functions. Including natural biology tools such as the "circadian clock" that regulate all brain sub-structures, the nervous system expresses its frustration as a progressive brain structural deterioration.


**Keywords:** sleep disturbance, sleep disorders, circadian clock, anxiety, stress, depression, sleep change patterns, neurological disorders, sleep/wake cycles, brain waves

## 1. Introduction

There are many conditions that can cause "sleep disturbance" for many different health conditions where "normal constant sleep" is interrupted since altering "falling asleep" to a "frequent disturbance for a long duration of time" usually implicit for a wide range of causes including environment alteration, health problems that affect physical or mental body functions, and others. Typically, the affected person with a "sleep disorder" tries to resolve the problem by paying attention to the "effect," and intending to avoid the disturbing conditions with temporal reachable solutions such as "traditional home remedies," that is, tea. If the situation continues, then they use "off-the-counter drugs" as sleep pills, that is, melatonin, and finally, when the situation is getting worse, they request professional medical help to find the "cause" of their unmanageable and possible "sleep disorder." Finding the cause of "sleep disturbance" and/or "sleep disorders" is not an easy task, even for medical professionals. In this time where humanity is confronting a huge amount of disasters due to "climate changes" with environmental changes that even have increased earth temperature, bacteria and viruses of different kinds have been evolving as a treat with a long pandemic time, and economic impacts do not present a near sign of stabilization; technological advances based on artificial intelligence that are making frequent changes in our way of living usually widen the amount of information that we receive and have to process. All these factors and many others are misdirecting the "basic survival need for the human being as amount and food, water, air quality, and the necessary and confronting need to sleep." All these facts have altered the pressure of the process and tried to find solutions to stabilize our situation, overusing our "brain and, by consequence, maximizing its normal functions." Including our natural biology tools, such as the "circadian clock," that regulate all the brain sub-structure is needed to process all the information and situations ASAP. Our nervous system by itself expresses its frustration as "progressive brain structural deterioration" generating different abnormal behaviors as "stress" (a physical, mental, and emotional factor), "anxiety" (an additional factor to stress reflecting as an emotion such as tension, excessive nervousness, fear, increased blood pressure), and many others as "depression."

All these factors are evolving into "sleep disorders," where frequently genetic factors are altered by "sleep change patterns" due to adjustments of shift of our own "circadian clock" by a big diversity of alteration as stress, and its response is detectable as anxiety and many others, including but not limited to aging, hormonal level changes, mood, sleep apnea, snoring, lifestyles, environment changes, restless leg syndrome, and many other reasons. If all these brain responses are not attended to, the possibility of permanent and destructive changes in our neuronal circuits can explain many abnormal behaviors in "neurological disorders" [1]. The research of all these factors is the main objective of this book chapter, "Sleep Medicine - Asleep or Awake."

## 2. Circadian clock, circadian rhythms, and physiological functions

The "circadian clock" is a biochemical oscillator clock or internal pacemaker in most living things that cycles with a stable phase and is synchronized with the solar time, It helps organisms and humans anticipate daily environmental changes of the day-night cycle and adjust their daily biology routines and behavior accordingly. "Circadian clock" is the central mechanism to drive "circadian rhythms." Some examples of circadian rhythms are sleep and wake cycles, hormonal activity, body temperature rhythm, eating, and digesting.

In humans, the "circadian clock" is slightly greater than 24 hours, and, earth's 24-hour rotation creates temporal variations, including light/dark cycles with temperature oscillations, which forces humans and other organisms to adapt to the cyclic environmental changes activate compensatory mechanisms and redundancy to maintain the function of the clock, providing "circadian rhythms," for many behaviors and physiological functions [2]: "sleep/wake cycle," "endocrine system," "metabolism," "immunity," and "mood." Where:

- The "sleep/wake cycle" is triggered by chemicals called "neurotransmitters" to send messages to different nerve cells in the brain to define "sleep/wake homeostasis," which handles the tendency to a relatively stable equilibrium between interdependent elements. The longer that we are awake, the greater our body senses the need to sleep at the end of the day, but our "circadian clock" causes highs and lows of sleepiness and wakefulness throughout the day. But plenty of regular sleep each night can help balance out these sleepy lows [3].

- The "endocrine system" is a network of glands in our body that make hormones to help cells talk to each other. A gland is an organ that makes and puts out hormones that do a specific job in your body. Endocrine and exocrine glands release the substances they make into your bloodstream, and they are responsible for almost every cell, organ, and function of our body by regulating the complexity of life in an organized way and other factors. The endocrine system is comprised of several glands. In many places in our body, including the human brain, there are three important glands:

    a. "hypothalamus," which connects your endocrine system with your nervous system.

    b. "Pituitary gland," which is attached to the "hypothalamus," indicates when the pituitary gland starts or stops making hormones, and

    c. "Pineal glands" make a chemical hormone called "melatonin" in response to darkness that helps your body get ready to go to sleep, and it has been linked to the regulation of circadian rhythms.

- "Metabolism" refers to the chemical processes that take place in our body to convert foods and drinks into energy. It is a complex process that combines calories and oxygen to create and release energy. This energy fuels body functions.

- "Immunity" is defined as the ability to resist infections or toxins by the action of antibodies or sensitized white blood cells.

- "Mood" is a temporary state of mind or feeling such as stress, anxiety, and many others. People who regularly experience mood swings are more likely to experience psychiatric disorders such as depression, anxiety, post-traumatic stress disorder, bipolar disorder, and borderline personality disorder. Mood swings in humans are likely caused in part by their genetics and their key developmental experiences, showing "high neuroticism," and they are just more likely to enter moods of anxiety and depression, particularly in response to stress [4].

**REMARK:** In a general way, we can say that if we alter the "circadian clock" as the central mechanism that drives "circadian rhythms," the alteration is reflected on the "sleep/wake homeostasis," driven by the "endocrine system" glands as the "hypothalamus" that connects the endocrine system with the nervous system, and is attached to the "pituitary gland," indicating when to start or stop making hormones. This alters the release of "melatonin" to initiate the normal "sleep cycle," and by consequence, this alters the release of "melatonin" to initiate the normal "sleep cycle," altering the nervous system that can be detected with "mood swing" showing as stress, anxiety, and other moods.

## 3. Brain waves and sleep stages

Our brain is always producing bursts of electrical activity identified as "electrical pulses" in the brain cell nerves known as "neurons." The "electrical pulses "are the way the neurons communicate to each other in their neuronal pathways to send orders or receive information, generating "wave activity" that can be detected and measured with a device known as an "electroencephalogram (EEG)" that evaluates the electric activity in the brain and records it in waves measured in cycles per second identified as "hertz (Hz)." Basically, the brain waves have a different speed from the fastest to the slowest frequency. There are five different types: gamma, beta, alpha, theta, and delta, as shown in **Table 1**.

"Sleep" is defined as the normal condition of body and mind, such as that which typically recurs for several hours every night, in which the nervous system is relatively inactive, the eyes are closed, the postural muscles are relaxed, and consciousness is practically suspended. The normal "sleep stages" are four, three of them with "non-rapid eye movements (NREM)" and one with "rapid eye movements (REM)" as indicated in **Table 1**, where the duration for each step is different at different ages.

- **Stage one, or N1 (sleep type NREM from 1 to 5 mins):** "Sleep" begins with a "lighter sleep" that can last from seconds up to 7 minutes, like a "short nap" where we can be easily woken, while the brain produces "alpha" and "theta" waves, and your eye movements slow down.

- **Stage two, or N2 (sleep type NREM from 10 to 60 mins):** It is also similar to a "light sleep" resembling a "larger nap," where we can wake up if we want. Here, if the brain produces a sudden increase in brain waves known as "sleep spindles," then the brain waves slow down.

| **Brain waves** | **Gamma** | **Beta** | **Alpha** | **Theta** | **Delta** |
|---|---|---|---|---|---|
| Frequency | Up to 100 Hz | 12–38 Hz | 8–12 Hz | 4–8 Hz | 0.5–4 Hz |
| Brain state<br>Sleep stage | Awake<br>Receptive and concentrated | Awake<br>Busy and focused | Awake to sleepy<br>Alert with calm awareness | Sleepy<br>Stages 1–2<br>N1 & N2<br>NREM | Deep sleep Stages 3<br>NREM & 4 REM |

**Table 1.**
*General brain wave types and brain states.*

- **Stage three, or N3, or slow-wave sleep (sleep type NREM from 20 to 40 mins):** It is the beginning of "deep sleep" and becomes a little harder to wake up because the body becomes less responsive to external stimulus. Here, the brain begins producing slower "delta waves" which are characterized by "no movement active in the eyes or muscles."

- **Stage four, or N4 (sleep type REM from 10 to 60 mins):** It moves to a "deeper sleep," and it is harder to wake up. Here, the brain is more active, producing more "delta waves" allowing a necessary "restorative stage," where the body repairs muscles, tissues, and tiny bone fractures, diminishes pain, stimulates growth and development, boosts immune function, and builds up energy for the next day.

Initially falling asleep, a "rapid eye movement (REM)" is observed, where the eyes make sudden movements in different directions, heart rate and blood pressure increase, and breathing becomes fast, irregular, and shallow. "REM" can last up to an hour, and an adult can have five or six of these cycles with intervals: "REM" and "non-rapid eye movement (NREM is also known as "progressive rapid eye movements (pREM))," where the brain consolidates and processes information from the day before so that it can be stored in your long-term memory; these "pREM intervals are very important to maintain the brain in good standing." Besides, "sleep spindles" are a type of brainwave that come in bursts, and they are described as an oscillatory activity of the brain that is mostly said to happen during stage 2, which is identified as "non-rapid eye movement NREM sleep," indicated as sleepy stages 1–2 in **Table 1**, and additionally occurs during deep sleep stages 3–4. "Sleep spindles" are described based on the frequency of waves as slow or fast: "slow spindles" occur between 9 and 12 Hz and originate in the frontal brain areas, and "fast spindles" have a range of 12 to 16 Hz from the central nervous system and peripheral parts.

> **REMARK**: The "circadian clock" generates the "sleep circadian rhythm" initiated by the release of "melatonin" for the "sleep cycle" that has four stages: in the first 2 from awake to sleepy generating "alpha" and "theta" brain waves, and in the last 2 with "deep sleep generating Delta" brain waves where the brain consolidates, and processes information accumulated during the day and moves from a short-term memory to a long-term memory through "pREM intervals" are very important to maintain the brain restored.

## 4. Introduction to neuroscience and circadian neuroscience

"Neuroscience" is the scientific study of the nervous system, including the brain, spinal cord, and peripheral nervous system, and its functions. "Circadian neuroscience" is a branch of neuroscience and chronobiology that looks at the neurological mechanisms that maintain "circadian rhythms" and investigates their subsequent effects on processes in the nervous system [5].

The human internal clock is controlled by the "Suprachiasmatic Nucleus (SCN)" located in a forward region of the brain area identified as the "hypothalamus" that connects your endocrine system with your nervous system, as explained in the last section. "SCN" contains a group of "neurons or nerve cells" that control the human body's "circadian rhythm." When the morning light is received by the eyes, an optical nerve senses it and sends the signal through neurons in the "SCN" that are sensitive to the light and release hormones such as "cortisol" that make an order for wake-up. At night, darkness is detected in the eyes, and the SCN sends a signal to the "pineal gland" that releases the chemical hormone that initiates the process of sleep, making our body feel sleepy [6].

## 5. Stress-anxiety take to sleep alteration

*"Stress"* is defined as a physical, mental, or emotional factor that causes bodily or mental tension. Stress can be external or internal. Where:

- External factors such as the environment, psychological, or social situations.
- Internal factors caused by illness, pain, or a medical procedure.

> **REMARK:** "Stress" is unavoidably something that everyone experiences throughout their lives. While some stress can pass quickly or feel acute, the most important thing is how we handle it.

"Anxiety" is an emotion characterized by feelings of tension, worried thoughts that lead to excessive nervousness, fear, apprehension, and inclusive physical symptoms such as increased blood pressure and others that may seriously affect day-to-day living.

> **REMARK:** "Anxiety" is the human brain's natural response to the "stress" accumulated.

Sleep alteration is an evolution of stress into anxiety, and this can be triggered by internal and external factors, as shown in **Figure 1**.

"Sleep Internal Alteration": Some frequent examples that cause "sleep change patterns" are: "inflammation," "injuries," "pain," "aging," "and other factors."

- "Inflammation" is a protective response of body tissues against stimuli such as pathogens, damaged cells, and irritants that are perceived as harmful.
- "Injuries" are defined as damages to the body caused by trauma by an external force or even internal factors such as inflammation.
- "Pain" is physical suffering or discomfort caused by illness or injury.
- "Aging" is generally accepted as an progressive function deterioration, and the "circadian clock" function and its rhythmic behavior decline, affecting the

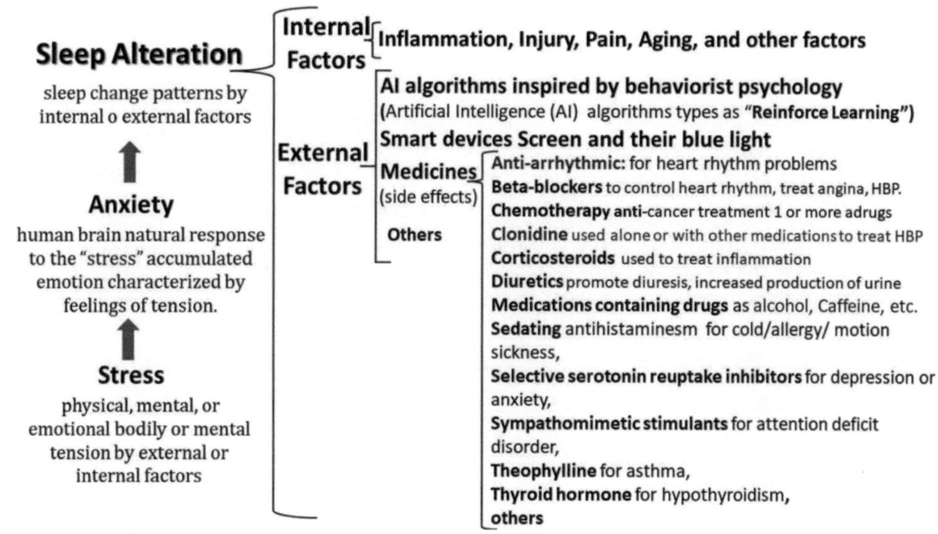


**Figure 1.**
*Sleep alteration is an evolution of the stress to anxiety, this can be triggered by internal and external factors as indicated.*

metabolism with changes such as glucose intolerance, nutrient sensing dysregulation, and mitochondrial dysfunction [2].

> **REMARK:** Aging body declination functions are reflected in metabolic disorders [7], such as obesity, diabetes, hypertension, and other changes that cause the human body to develop "sleep disorders."

"Sleep external alteration" examples that cause "sleep change patterns" could be in many ways, the most common are "artificial intelligence algorithms inspired by behaviorist psychology," "smart device screens and their blue light," and prescribed medicine side effects." Where:

- "Artificial Intelligence algorithms inspired by behaviorist psychology apps such as email, chats, text, social networking, running on all smart devices that we use every day as: mobile phones, tablets, computers, etc. These apps constantly make interruptions to alter our natural behaviors applying AI algorithms as "reinforce learning" that are deigned to keep our attention constantly by activities based on rewards of different types with the purpose of creating addiction on us for different purposes from statistics, commercial, political, etc., for example:
    - "Search engines online" such as Google, Microsoft Bing, Yahoo, Baidu, Ask.com, and many more to search information on webpages, images, news, research papers, books, etc.
    - "Social media," such as Instagram, Facebook, Snapchat, Twitter, TikTok, YouTube, and many others, are controlling the lives of their users. On a daily basis, they frequently control users by checking their notifications and

sighing in dissatisfaction because they have not gotten enough likes on your profile picture or comments.

- "News websites" are always updating, generating, and adding new news to meet the need to be informed. These websites analyze the traffic and your activities and, with statistics, detect what is of more general interest, and if they have your username, they personalize the news for them, to maintain their attention and force them to check frequently for updates that are important for them, such as stock prices, public health, to accomplish user awareness.

> **REMARK:** "Artificial intelligence algorithms inspired by behaviorist psychology" running on smart devices create "addiction," which is handled by the need to stay up-to-date to try to relax the anxiety generated by "stress." The main problem is that we expend part of our energy on unimportant things that do not benefit our important daily duties, at the end of the day, we feel more nervous, and these thoughts alter our daily sleep [8].

- "Smart devices Screen and their blue light." The problem with the display on smart devices LED (light-emitting diode) flat panel that emits blue light beside others from small displays and more large-scale video displays. It uses an array of LED units known as modules, consisting of many small LED chips placed on a printed circuit board (PCB) substrate. On a natural rainbow, we see the visual light spectrum; these are the colors visible to the human eye and include red, blue, and green "wavelengths." All light we see is a combination of these wavelengths, including light from the sun and exposure to blue light from the sun as well as our screens, which boost mood and alertness, that is, sunrise signals to our brain that it is time to wake up. In the evening, these flat screens can disrupt "our body's natural sleep cycle," known as the "circadian rhythm," which synchronizes the "sleep-awake cycle" with night and day. By slowing the natural production of "melatonin." It is a natural hormone that is produced by the "pineal gland in the brain" and then released into the bloodstream to make us follow the natural "circadian rhythm" cycle [9].

> **REMARK:** Almost everyone has an occasional night with little or low-quality sleep. But when sleep problems start to affect your "quality of life," you may develop a "sleep disorder." The most common sleep disorder caused by too much exposure to "smart device screen blue light" is "insomnia," which refers to habitual sleeplessness, and it is the most common "sleep disorder" in the world. Besides, "insomnia" is more common as you get older, and it can affect your life in a number of ways, including daytime fatigue, poor concentration, and low mood.

- "Medicines side effects": many of them may cause "sleep deprivation" as "anti-arrhythmic," "beta-blockers" for high blood pressure, or heart rhythm problems or angina; "chemotherapy" for cancer; "clonidine" for high blood pressure; "corticosteroids" for inflammation or asthma; "diuretics" for high blood pressure; "medications containing drugs" as headaches or pain relievers; "sedating antihistamines" for cold, allergy, or motion sickness; "selective serotonin reuptake inhibitors" for depression or anxiety; "sympathomimetic stimulants" for attention deficit disorder; "theophylline" for asthma; "thyroid hormone" for hypothyroidism, and many others [10].

- "Anti-arrhythmic" for heart rhythm problems There are four classes of antiarrhythmics, based on the Vaughan-Williams (VW) classification system [11]:

    a. Class I sodium channel blockers to slow electrical impulses in heart muscles include disopyramide, flecainide, mexiletine, propafenone, and quinidine.

    b. Class II beta blockers slow down the heart rate, often by blocking hormones such as adrenaline. that is, acebutolol, atenolol, bisoprolol, metoprolol, nadolol, and propranolol.

    c. Class III potassium channel blockers slow down electrical impulses in all of the heart's cells, that is, amiodarone, bretylium, dofetilide, dronedarone, ibutilide, and sotalol.

    d. Class IV, nondihydropyridine calcium channel blockers to decrease heart rate and contractions, such as diltiazem and verapamil,

    e. Other antiarrhythmic drugs not included in the VW classification are adenosine, digoxin, and blood thinners.

- "Beta-blockers" to control heart rhythm, treat angina, and reduce high blood pressure, that is, Acebutolol, Atenolol, Betaxolol, Bisoprolol (Zebeta, Ziac) Carteolol, Carvedilol, Labetalol (Normodyne, Trandate).

- "Chemotherapy" is a type of cancer treatment that uses one or more anticancer drugs as chemotherapeutic agents, alkylating agents, or others [12]. It is important to know that not all medicines and drugs to treat cancer work the same way. Other drugs to treat cancer work differently, such as "targeted therapy," "hormone therapy," and "immunotherapy."

- "Clonidine" is used alone or with other medications to treat high blood pressure (hypertension). Brand Names: Catapres-TTS-2; Catapres-TTS-3; Catapres-TTS-1.

- "Corticosteroids" are any group of steroid hormones produced in the adrenal cortex or made synthetically. There are two kinds: glucocorticoids and mineralocorticoids. They have various metabolic functions, and some are used to treat inflammation. Some corticosteroid medicines include cortisone, prednisone, and methylprednisolone. Prednisone is the most commonly used type of steroid to treat certain rheumatologic diseases (like rheumatoid arthritis or lupus) [13].

- "Diuretics" are substances that promote diuresis, the increased production of urine, helping rid the body of salt (sodium) and water. Help your kidneys release more sodium into your urine. The sodium helps remove water from your blood, decreasing the amount of fluid flowing through your veins and arteries. This reduces blood pressure. As shown in [14].

a. Thiazide types include chlorothiazide, chlorthalidone, hydrochlorothiazide, indapamide, and metolazone.

b. Loop type: bumetanide (Bumex), ethacrynic acid (Edecrin), furosemide (Lasix), and torsemide (Soaanz).

c. Potassium sparing types include bumetanide (Bumex), ethacrynic acid (Edecrin), furosemide (lasix), torsemide (Soaanz).

- "Medications containing drugs" for different purposes as headaches or pain relievers include "alcohol" (for cough, cold, and flu), "caffeine" (for headaches and other pain), "nicotine replacement" (avoid smoking), and others.
- "Sedating antihistamines" for colds, allergies, or motion sickness,
- "Selective serotonin reuptake inhibitors" for depression or anxiety,
- "Sympathomimetic stimulants" for attention deficit disorder,
- "Theophylline" for asthma,
- "Thyroid hormone" for hypothyroidism,
- and many others.

**REMARK:** If prescribed medicines are affecting your "sleep pattern," it is strongly recommended to inform your healthcare provider to correct this issue ASAP.

**IMPORTANT:** Never take medicine for sleep without a medical prescription and follow-up medical supervision.

## 6. Sleep-wake and circadian disorders and neurological disorders

"Central nervous system (CNS)" lesions appear by disrupting continuously the "sleep-wake cycle" based on constant alteration of the human "circadian clock" developing into "circadian disorders." These are identified as "sleep-wake and circadian disorders (SWCD)," leading primary to lesioning specific cell types or structures generating or regulating sleep, wake, and circadian functions or through nonspecific lesioning of diffuse neural networks. In addition, "SWCD" can arise secondarily from complications of "CNS" lesions such as spasticity, "muscle stiffness and spasms," "pain," and even "depression."

As explained in Section: Introduction to Neuroscience and Circadian Neuroscience, "Circadian rhythms" signals from the "Suprachiasmatic Nucleus (SCN)" are distributed in the brain and the entire body by two main cell-brain connections identified as pathways: the "Hormonal rhythms control pathway" and the "Euro humoral pathway" [15]. These are:

1. "Hormonal rhythms control pathways" transmitted by terminals of the SCN from the brain to organs with the release of neurotransmitters and a group of them known as "neuropeptides" [16].

2. "Euro humoral pathway" involving secretion of diffusible output signals regulating preferentially the rest-activity rhythm as: heart rate, muscular strength, insulin, leptin, and glycemia. Where:

    a. "Heart rate rhythm" is a healthy "sinoatrial (SA) node" a special cardiac muscle in the upper back wall of the right atrium made up of cells known as "pacemaker cells." It has an intrinsic heartbeat generation rate of 60 to 80. If the atrium fails to generate a heartbeat, then a healthy "atrioventricular node (AV)" can do so at a rate of about 40, and if needed, the ventricles themselves can generate heartbeats at a rate of about 20 per minute.

    b. "Muscular strength rhythm" is the "circadian rhythm" in muscle force that has also been described for maximal dynamic contractions and isometric contractions. The "acrophase" (time of the maximal level of the rhythm) of the muscle capacity to develop maximal force has been found in the evening compared with the morning. The diurnal variations in muscle performance can be influenced by several factors, such as core temperature, sleep deprivation, warm-up duration, and hormone concentrations such as cortisol and catecholamine [17].

    c. "Insulin rhythm": levels of both insulin and the counterregulatory hormones, which work against the action of insulin, are influenced by a "circadian rhythm." The counterregulatory hormones, which include glucagon, epinephrine (adrenaline), growth hormone, and cortisol, raise blood glucose levels when needed [18].

    d. "Leptin rhythm," where leptin is a pleiotropic protein hormone produced mainly by fat cells, regulates metabolic activity and many other physiological functions. The intrinsic circadian rhythm of blood leptin is modulated by gender, development, feeding, fasting, sleep, obesity, and endocrine disorders [19]

    e. "Glycemia rhythm" refers to the concentration of sugar or glucose in the blood. Glycemia is measured by a number called the glycemic index, which reflects how much an individual's blood sugar level rises after consuming 50 grams of carbohydrate compared with someone without diabetes who has consumed 50 grams of carbohydrate.

In many cases, the "sleep-wake and circadian disorders" may worsen over time, leading primary to lesioning specific cell types or structures on the brain. That could present the first manifestations of an underlying neurologic disorder such as "dream enactment behavior in Parkinson disease (PD)," "excessive daytime sleepiness (EDS) in hypothalamic disorders," or "insomnia in Alzheimer disease (AD)" [20]. Finally, through time it is evolving as an identifiable "progressive neurologic disease."

> **REMARK:** The brain is the one that drives sleep and wakefulness through the "circadian clock," which acts as a natural pacemaker, adjusting our daily lives with day-night based on the detection of solar light, allowing us to do our routines and behaviors that are driven by "circadian rhythms." Their continuous alterations are reflected in "sleep-wake and circadian disorders," which sooner or later affect neural brain networks, memory, circadian preferences, neural development, and unresponsiveness to outside events. All these changes are ways to develop and could be associated with "progressive neurologic diseases" with abnormalities such as insomnia, schizophrenia, epilepsy, mental retardation, and mental health issues observed in Parkinson's, Alzheimer's, and other diseases.

## 7. How to analyze sleep-wake and circadian disorders

The "sleep-wake-circadian pathologies" are generally underdiagnosed in neurologic patients despite their major impact on the onset, evolution, and outcome of neurodevelopmental disorders in the sense of an illness that disrupts normal physical or mental functions, including attention-deficit hyperactivity disorder (ADHD), autism spectrum disorders (ASDs), Prader-Willi syndrome (PWS), and Smith-Magenis syndrome (SMS), and diseases as progressive disorders with abnormal conditions that negatively affect the structure or function of all or part of an organism, and that is not immediately due to any external or internal injury, such as Parkinson's, Alzheimer, and many more. The main key in this research paper is to focus on accessible technologies and methodologies that are necessary for the periodic evaluation of "sleep-wake and circadian disorders." These are summarized in **Figure 2**. With the purpose of measuring the progression effect or efficacy of their therapeutic interventions and helping to evaluate the progression of "sleep-wake and circadian disorders" that could lead to neurologic disorders and diseases, separated on four instrument types: "personal home monitor," "lab studying testing," and "neuroimaging."

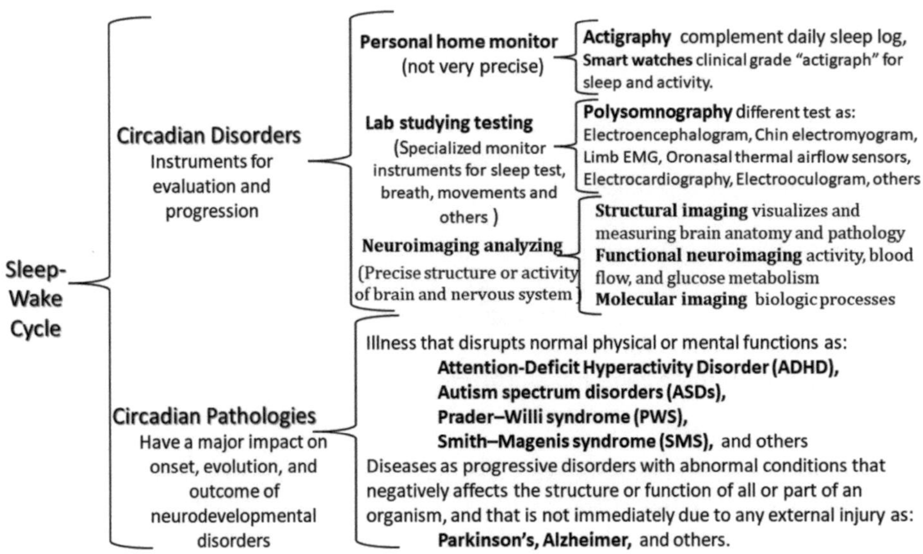


**Figure 2.**
*Sleep-wake cycle circadian disorders instruments for evaluation of progression and sleep-wake cycle circadian pathologies.*

- "Personal home monitors" are devices characterized for their low cost, allowing personal home sleep monitors to:

    - "Actigraphy" or "actometer" is worn on the nondominant wrist or ankle to record acceleration or deceleration of body movements. It is worn for days or weeks and complements a daily sleep log for the diagnostic "circadian rhythm sleep disorders" and other primary sleep disorders such as insomnia and idiopathic hypersomnia.

    - "Smart watches." Today, some smart watches include a clinical-grade "actigraph" used for sleep and activity home monitoring, showing an easy-to-follow and understand graph with automatic daily recordings, with high accuracy and sensitivity, very useful as primary personal feedback, that allows you to take the information collected to the medical doctor with valid information on your personal "sleep/wake cycle" for an initial diagnostic of "circadian rhythm sleep disorders." Please be sure to buy a clinically validated smart watch for sleep monitoring [21].

- "Labs studying testing" are labs studying combining specialized monitor instruments for evaluation of sleep tests, breathing, movements, and others based on specialized medical instruments that must be handled by specialized people to place the sensor and run the test as specified by medical specifications using a diversity of them defined in general as "Polysomnography" [22]:

    - "Electroencephalogram (EEG)" to measure electrical activity in the brain using electrodes attached to the scalp, for detecting and analyzing several polygraphic physiologies during sleep.

    - "Chin electromyogram (EMG)" to assess the health of muscles and the nerve cells that control the chin and allow determination of sleep stages.

    - "Limb EMG" for leg muscle evaluation, detecting and analyzing periodic leg movements that may disrupt sleep as "restless legs syndrome," and other evaluations.

    - "Oronasal thermal airflow sensors" use thermistors or thermocouples to measure and analyze thermal airflow, reading the difference between the temperature of exhaled and ambient air to estimate airflow and detect mouth breathing. Interrupt during sleep as "sleep apnea," and other issues.

    - "Electrocardiography" is the process of producing an electrocardiogram (ECG or EKG) recording the heart's electrical activity.

    - "Electrooculogram" for measuring the cornea-retinal standing potential that exists between the front and the back of the human eye and detection of eye movements.

    - And many other instruments, such as "pulse oximetry" for measuring arterial oxygen saturation and "audiovisual recordings," enhance the diagnostic utility of polysomnography.

"Polysomnography" is used to diagnose sleep-disordered breathing, movement disorders, and abnormal behavior during sleep, such as "REM sleep behavior disorder" and arousal disorders.

> **REMARK:** "Polysomnography" is very useful to analyze the sleep architecture process for the wakefulness stage, Stage W, and NREM and REM sleep stages, as shown in **Table 1**.

- "Neuroimaging analyzing" is the process of producing images of the structure or activity of the brain or other part of the nervous system by biomedical instruments such as "magnetic resonance imaging (MIR)" or "computerized tomography (CT)" and other neuroimaging technologies. Neuroimaging approaches can be broadly divided into three types:
    - "Structural imaging," which visualizes brain anatomy and pathology and measures volume and other tissue characteristics,
    - "Functional neuroimaging," measuring brain activity, blood flow, and glucose metabolism; and
    - "Molecular imaging" focuses on information on biologic processes, including protein aggregation, neuroinflammation, and related processes.

The development of "functional neuroimaging" consists of all techniques that can generate images of brain activity. In humans, such techniques usually include "single photon emission computed tomography (SPECT)," "positron emission tomography (PET)," "functional magnetic resonance imaging (fMRI)," "optical imaging," "diffusion tensor imaging (DTI)," "multichannel electroencephalography (EEG)," "magnetoencephalography (MEG)," and others. Each technique has its own advantages and drawbacks in terms of spatial and temporal resolution, accessibility, safety, and cost [23]. Applying AI algorithms detected following:

- "Sleep-wake cycle," detecting brain activity throughout the brain in this cycle.
    - "Regional brain activity" identifies them when they are influenced by incoming stimuli as well as by previous waking experience.
    - "Neural correlates of sleep-wake regulation tend toward a relatively stable equilibrium between interdependent elements for sleep pressure and the non-visual effect of light."
    - "Functional imaging of patients with sleep disorders: studying their neural system changes across the sleep-awake cycle."

Many researchers applying "neuroimaging techniques" have discovered the relation of the "sleep-wake cycle" with neurological diseases such as: "REM sleep behavior disorder," "isolated rapid eye movement (REM) sleep behavior disorder," "type 2 diabetes mellitus and sleep disorders,"

- "REM sleep behavior disorder (RBD)" may be idiopathic or associated with other neurologic disorders, and there is a strong association between RBD and "α-synucleinopathy" which are neurodegenerative diseases characterized by the abnormal accumulation of aggregates of alpha-synuclein protein in neurons, nerve fibers, or glial cells. They have observed groups for sleep disorders and signs at the clinical onset of neurodegenerative disease by studying and comparing structural and functional MRI to identify brain changes that progress over time in patients [24].

- "Isolated rapid eye movement (REM) sleep behavior disorder (iRBD)" was detected in patients with neurology symptoms of "Mild Cognitive Impairment (MCI)" presenting long-term verbal memory and visuospatial functions, as well as attentional-executive impairment "reduced cerebral glucose consumption in brain areas critical for cognition" and a more severe deafferentation of the "nigro-striatal" regions in the brain. Then, there is the importance of identifying iRBD patients with MCI for urgent neuroprotective trials [25]. "Wakefulness" is associated mainly with the following brain structures: the frontal and parietal polymodal associative cortices.

- "Type 2 diabetes mellitus (T2DM) and sleep disorders (SD)" are both common diseases related to brain functional and structural abnormalities involving the "hypothalamic-pituitary-adrenal (HPA)" axis. "T2DM" is a chronic metabolic and inflammatory disease accompanied by insulin resistance, hyperglycemia, and defective insulin secretion from the pancreas. All included studies showed that alternative interventions improved sleep quality, glucose levels, blood lipids, hypertension, and weight management, but whether acupuncture and other alternative treatments for long-term T2DM and SD can decrease disease-associated risks and complications is yet to be determined. Sleep disturbances in T2DM patients are related to the brain organs, and "obesity" manifests with sleep problems as "insomnia."

    - "Obesity," Neuroimaging analysis demonstrated that there were altered interactions in the brain networks of obese individuals in response to food cues [26], particularly in the frontal-mesolimbic network [27].

    - In "insomnia," the main affected brain areas are the "ascending reticular activating system," "hippocampus," "amygdala," "insular cortex," and "medial prefrontal cortices" [28].

"Molecular Imaging (MI)" is a growing biomedical research discipline that enables the visualization, characterization, and quantification of biologic processes taking place at the cellular and subcellular levels within intact living patients in their own psychological environment. Examples of progressive neurologic diseases are "Parkinson's disease," "Alzheimer's disease," "frontotemporal dementia," "multiple system atrophy," and many more related to disturbances in the "sleep/wake cycle."

- "Parkinson's disease (PD)" in patients has a high degree of sleep problems, one of "two common accumulations of proteins" related to different types of Parkinson's identified as "idiopathy Parkinson's," the most common at about 85%, and "atypical Parkinson's," the least common at about 15% [29]. Both types of "PD" have a bidirectional relationship with sleep through the accumulation of proteins in the neuron cells: "α-synuclein" and "Tau."

    - "α-synuclein or synuclein alpha" is also known by the alias "SNCA or NACP or PARK1 or PARK4 or PD1." "α-synuclein" is a neuronal protein that regulates synaptic vesicle trafficking and subsequent neurotransmitter release. It is abundant in the brain, mainly in the axon terminals of presynaptic neurons, and

    - "Tau or tubulin," also known by the alias "MAPT (microtubule-associated protein tau) or DDPAC or FTDP-17 or MAPTL or MSTD or MTBT1 or MTBT2 or PPND or PPP1R103 or microtubule-associated protein tau ortau-40," is a group of six highly soluble protein isoforms produced by alternative splicing from the gene MAPT. They have roles primarily in maintaining the stability of microtubules in axons and are abundant in the neurons of the "central nervous system (CNS)," where the cerebral cortex has the highest abundance. It is found in atypical Parkinson's known as "Progressive Supranuclear Palsy," which often shows "midbrain" and "superior cerebellar peduncular atrophy" and cell loss in a specific distribution, particularly affecting the "subthalamic nucleus," "globus pallidus," "substantia nigra," and "pretectal area of the midbrain" [30].

- "Alzheimer's disease (AD)" is the most prevalent neurodegenerative disorder and the most common cause of dementia with abnormal "tau protein accumulation." Disturbances of the "sleep/wake" cycle in "AD" are very common, frequently precede cognitive decline, and tend to worsen with disease progression. "Sleep-wake cycles" are regulated by neuromodulator centers located in the "brainstem," "hypothalamus," and "basal forebrain," many of which are vulnerable to the accumulation of abnormal protein deposits associated with neurodegenerative conditions. There is evidence that "tau" protein accumulation-driven neuropathology is a primary driver of sleep disturbance in AD [31].

- "Frontotemporal dementia (FTD)" is the second most common cause of young-onset dementia. Our understanding of FTD and its related syndromes has advanced significantly in recent years. Among the most prominent areas of progress is the overlap between FTD, motor neuron diseases (MND), and other neurodegenerative conditions at a clinicopathologic and genetic level. There is emerging evidence that "hypothalamic" dysfunction, manifesting as disturbances in sleep and metabolism, is an integral component of neurodegeneration [32].

- "Multiple system atrophy (MSA)" is a sporadic and progressive neurodegenerative disorder characterized by abnormal "α-synuclein" aggregation in oligodendroglia and neuronal loss in multiple areas of the central nervous system, and many report sleep-related breathing disorders as inspiratory sighs that are considered a diagnostic red flag for the parkinsonian form of MSA [33].

And many other neurologic diseases usually present sleep disturbances.

**REMARKS:** Sleep and mental health are closely connected. Sleep deprivation affects our psychological state and mental health. And they are particularly common in patients with anxiety, depression, bipolar disorder, and attention deficit hyperactivity disorder, and also have connections with neurologic disease.

## 8. Conclusions and comments

"Sleep quality" is critical for the maintenance of a stable equilibrium of body function driven by "circadian function," especially for "neuronal cells and pathways" in the brain, endocrine system, metabolism, immunity, and others. If we leave unattended the importance of normal "sleep/wake cycles," our human body is taken to the next step, presenting "chronic sleep disturbances" through the increment of undesirable "mood swings," presenting symptoms of stress, anxiety, and many others. People who regularly experience "mood swings" are more likely to experience "psychiatric disorders" such as "anxiety," "depression," "post-traumatic stress disorder," "bipolar disorder," and "borderline personality disorder." And with time, the same situations grow to have significant "cognitive" and "physical health" consequences that likely exacerbate disease severity as "neurological disorders." Today, there are technologies that can detect and evaluate "sleep-wake and circadian disorders," measuring and tracking the severity of the damage with "specialized lab tests," such as "polysomnography," that combine specialized monitor instruments for evaluation of sleep tests, breathing, movements, and others. Technologic advances based on "neuroimaging analyzing," "functional neuroimaging," and "molecular imaging" that allow the discovery of new "genetic mutations" as well as the development of "potential biomarkers" may serve to further expand knowledge to help with "sleep quality" that is affecting millions of people and continues growing around the world.

The odds of being "sleep deprived with less than 6 hours a night for adults" have increased significantly over the past 30 years as the lines between work and home have become blurred and digital technology has firmly become part of our lifestyles [34].

**FINAL REMARK:** "Sleep quality" is affecting millions of people and continues to grow around the world. Today, there are technologies that can detect and evaluate "sleep-wake and circadian disorders" before they cause chaos on our neuronal circuits, creating endless multiple neurologic responses that could take us to "degenerative diseases that still have no cure."

Please sleep well.
Thanks.
Dr. Jorge Garza- Ulloa.
More information: https://garzaulloa.org

Notices: Knowledge and best practice in this field are constantly changing as new research and experience broaden our understanding, and changes in research methods, professional practices, or medical treatment may become necessary. To the fullest extent of the law, neither the publisher nor the authors, contributors, or editors, assume any liability for any injury and/or damage to persons or property as a matter of products liability, negligence, or otherwise, or from any use or operation of any methods, products, instructions, or ideas contained in the material herein.

## Author details

Jorge Garza-Ulloa
Research Consulting Service, El Paso, Texas, USA

*Address all correspondence to: jorge@garzaulloa.org

## References

[1] Garza-Ulloa J. Theory of stress-anxiety-sleep disorders-neural damage cyclic chain and the progression of Parkinson's disease. American Journal of Biomedical Science & Research. 2019;**6**(3). AJBSR.MS.ID.001021. DOI: 10.34297/AJBSR.2019.06.001021

[2] Sato S, Solanas G, Sassone-Corsi P, Benitah SA. Tuning up an aged clock: Circadian clock regulation in metabolism and aging. Translational Medicine of Aging. 2022;**6**:1-13. ISSN 2468-5011. DOI: 10.1016/j.tma.2021.11.003

[3] Hopkins J. Sleep/wake cycle. Available from: https://www.hopkinsmedicine.org/health/conditions-and-diseases/sleepwake-cycles [accessed 12/3/2022]

[4] Lilienfeld SO, Andrews BP. Development, and preliminary validation of a self-report measure of psychopathic personality traits in noncriminal populations. Journal of Personality Assessment. 1996;**66**:488-524

[5] Available from: https://en.wikipedia.org/wiki/Neuroscience#cite_note-Merriam-1 [accessed 12/3/2022]

[6] Available from: https://www.hopkinsmedicine.org/health/conditions-and-diseases/sleepwake-cycles [accessed 12/3/2022]

[7] Hernandez-Segura A, Nehme J, Demaria M. Hallmarks of cellular senescence. Trends in Cell Biology. 2018;**28**(6):436-453

[8] Garza-Ulloa J. The healthy balance between natural and artificial intelligence. Novel Research in Sciences 2002;**12**(4). NRS.000794. DOI: 10.31031/NRS.2022.12.000794

[9] Available from: https://www.aao.org/eye-health/tips-prevention/digital-devices-your-eyes,11/3/2022 [accessed 12/3/2022]

[10] Available from: https://www.sleepstation.org.uk/articles/medicines/medicines-that-can-affect-sleep/#:~:text=Medications%20that%20may%20interfere%20with%20sleep%20%20,High%20blood%20pressure%20%2010%20more%20rows%20 [accessed 12/3/2022]

[11] Available from: https://my.clevelandclinic.org/health/drugs/22867-what-are-antiarrhythmics [accessed 4/16/2023]

[12] Available from: https://www.cancer.org/treatment/treatments-and-side-effects/treatment-types/chemotherapy/how-chemotherapy-drugs-work.html [accessed 4/16/2023]

[13] Available from: https://my.clevelandclinic.org/health/drugs/4812-corticosteroids [accessed 4/16/2023]

[14] Available from: https://www.mayoclinic.org/diseases-conditions/high-blood-pressure/in-depth/diuretics/art-20048129 [accessed 4/16/2023]

[15] Edith G, Etienne C. Chapter 38 - central and peripheral circadian clocks. In: Meir K, Thomas R, Dement William C, editors. Principles and Practice of Sleep Medicine. Sixth ed. Elsevier; 2017. pp. 396-404.e6. ISBN 9780323242882. Available from: https://www.sciencedirect.com/science/article/pii/B9780323242882000386

[16] Meyer-Bernstein EL, Jetton AE, Matsumoto SI, et al. Effects of suprachiasmatic transplants on circadian rhythms of neuroendocrine function in golden hamsters. Endocrinology. 1999;**140**:207-218

[17] Zbidi S, Zinoubi B, Vandewalle H, Driss T. Diurnal rhythm of muscular strength depends on temporal specificity of self-resistance training. Journal of Strength and Conditioning Research. 2016;**30**(3):717-724. DOI: 10.1519/JSC.0000000000001144

[18] Available from: https://www.diabetesselfmanagement.com/diabetes-resources/definitions/circadian-rhythm/#:~:text=Circadian%20Rhythm.%20Levels%20of%20both%20insulin%20and%20the,and%20cortisol%2C%20raise%20blood%20glucose%20levels%20when%20needed [accessed 12/3/2022]

[19] Pan W, Kastin AJ. Leptin: A biomarker for sleep disorders? Sleep Medicine Reviews. 2014;**18**(3):283-290. DOI: 10.1016/j.smrv.2013.07.003. Epub 2013 Sep 27

[20] Schmidt MH, Dekkers MPJ, Baillieul S, Jendoubi J, Wulf M-A, Wenz E, et al. Measuring sleep, wakefulness, and circadian functions in neurologic disorders, Sleep Medicine Clinics. 2021; **16**(4):661-671. ISSN 1556-407X. ISBN 9780323897600. DOI: 10.1016/j.jsmc.2021.08.005

[21] Roomkham S, Hittle M, Cheung J, et al. Sleep monitoring with the apple watch: Comparison to a clinically validated actigraph [version 1; peer review: 2 approved with reservations, 1 not approved]. F1000Research. 2019;**8**: 754. DOI: 10.12688/f1000research.19020.1

[22] Nofzinger EA, Maquet P. Chapter 12 - what brain imaging reveals about sleep generation and maintenance. In: Kryger M, Roth T, Dement WC, editors. Principles and Practice of Sleep Medicine. Sixth ed. 2017; Elsevier: pp. 118-131.e4. ISBN 80323242882. DOI: 10.1016/B978-0-323-24288-2.00012-X. Available from: https://www.sciencedirect.com/science/article/pii/B978032324288200012X

[23] Risacher SL, Saykin AJ. Chapter 12 - neuroimaging in aging and neurologic diseases. In: Dekosky ST, Asthana S, editors. Handbook of Clinical Neurology. Vol. 167. Elsevier. Available from: https://www.sciencedirect.com/science/article/pii/B9780128047668000121

[24] Ferini-Strambi L. Does idiopathic REM sleep behavior disorder (iRBD) really exist? What are the potential markers of neurodegeneration in iRBD? Sleep Medicine. 2011;**12**(Suppl 2):S43-S49. DOI: 10.1016/j.sleep.2011.10.010

[25] Vacca M, Assogna F, et al. Neuropsychiatric, neuropsychological, and neuroimaging features in isolated REM sleep behavior disorder: The importance of MCI. Sleep Medicine. 2022;**100**:230-237. ISSN 1389-9457. DOI: 10.1016/j.sleep.2022.08.018 Available from: https://www.sciencedirect.com/science/article/pii/S1389945722011236

[26] Ding Y, Ji G, Li G, et al. Altered interactions among resting-state networks in individuals with obesity. Obesity. 2020;**28**(3):601-608. DOI: 10.1002/oby.22731

[27] Meng Q, Han Y, Ji G, et al. Disrupted topological organization of the frontal-mesolimbic network in obese patients. Brain Imaging and Behavior. 2018;**12**(6): 1544-1555. DOI: 10.1007/s11682-017-9802-z

[28] von Deneen KM, Garstka MA. Neuroimaging perspective in targeted treatment for type 2 diabetes melitus and sleep disorders. Intelligent Medicine. 2022;**2**(4):209-220. ISSN 2667-1026. DOI: 10.1016/j.imed.2022.05.003. Available from: https://www.sciencedirect.com/science/article/pii/S2667102622000390

[29] Jorge Garza-Ulloa. Update on Parkinson's disease. American Journal of Biomedical Science & Research. 2019;**2** (6). AJBSR.MS.ID.000614. DOI: 10.34297/AJBSR.2019.02.000614

[30] Morris HR. Chapter 21 - progressive Supranuclear palsy. In: Schapira AHV, Lang AET, Fahn S, editors. Blue Books of Neurology. Vol. 34. Butterworth-Heinemann; 2010. pp. 361-374. ISSN 1877-184X. ISBN 9781416066415. DOI: 10.1016/B978-1-4160-6641-5.00021-0. Available from: https://www.sciencedirect.com/science/article/abs/pii/B9781416066415000210

[31] Lew CH, Petersen C, Neylan TC, Grinberg LT. Tau-driven degeneration of sleep- and wake-regulating neurons in Alzheimer's disease. Sleep Medicine Reviews. 2021;**60**:101541. ISSN 1087-0792. DOI: 10.1016/j.smrv.2021.10154

[32] Hwang YT, Piguet O, Hodges JR, Grunstein R, Burrell JR. Sleep and orexin: A new paradigm for understanding behavioural-variant frontotemporal dementia? Sleep Medicine Reviews. 2020;**54**:101361. ISSN 1087-0792. DOI: 10.1016/j.smrv.2020.101361

[33] Parreira S, Antunes F, Coelho M, Bentes C, Peralta R. Sighs during sleep in multiple system atrophy. Sleep Medicine. 2021;**78**:75-80. ISSN 1389-9457. DOI: 10.1016/j.sleep.2020.12.013

[34] sleephealth.org. Available from: https://www.sleephealth.org/sleep-health/the-state-of-sleephealth-in-america/#:~:text=It%20is%20estimated%20that%20sleep-related%20problems%20affect%2050,been%20identified%20in%20minorities%20and%20underserved%20populations.%202 [accessed 12/3/2022]

Section 2

# Evaluation and Management – Asleep or Awake

Chapter 4

# Clinical Assessment of Children and Young People with Sleep Problems and Co-Morbid Neurodevelopmental Disorders

*Michael O. Ogundele, Chinnaiah Yemula and Hani F. Ayyash*


## Abstract

Sleep disorders are very common among children and young people (CYP) with neurodevelopmental, emotional, behavioural and intellectual disorders (NDEBID). NDEBID include several conditions such as Attention Deficit/Hyperactivity Disorder (ADHD), Autism Spectrum Disorder (ASD), Cerebral palsy (CP), Epilepsy and Learning (Intellectual) disorders. Extant literature have reported up to 80% of CYP with NDEBID experiencing different types of chronic insomnia, compared to 3–36% of their otherwise normally developing counterparts. Sleep disorders among CYP with NDEBID have severe negative consequences on the affected individuals and their families. Chronic sleep deprivation causes behavioural, memory and attention problems, mood disorders, impaired cognitive development, learning abilities, and school performances. It also significantly increases the stress level and impact the wellbeing of other family members and impair family cohesion. Sleep disorders therefore further aggravate both internalising and externalising behaviours, emotional wellbeing and daily functioning of CYP with NDEBID. This chapter provides a brief summary of the various important aspects of sleep physiology, aetiology, classification and prevalence of sleep disorders among CYP with NDEBIDs. It outlines various behavioural, non-pharmacological management strategies and pharmacotherapy. Practical tips for clinicians are outlined in an easy-to read flow chart, including sections on assessment, investigations, care plan formulation and follow-up.


**Keywords:** sleep, emotional, neurodevelopmental disorders, pharmacotherapy, non-pharmacologic interventions, cognitive therapy, insomnia, melatonin, children, adolescents, psychoeducation

## 1. Introduction

Sleep problems affects all age group of children from preschool age to adolescence, with a prevalence of up to 80% reported among children and young people (CYP) with Neurodevelopmental (and related Neurodisability), Emotional, Behavioural, Intellectual and Disorders (NDEBID). This is disproportionately higher than the prevalence of 3–36% among typically developing children and adolescents [1, 2].

The prevalence of sleep disorders in CYP with NDEBID is also related to the degree of their disability. For example the prevalence of sleep disorders among adolescents with learning disability varies between 26% for moderate disability to 44% for severe disability. This compares with prevalence of 15–19% among adolescents with no disability [1].

Sleep disorders among CYP with NDEBID have severe negative consequences on the affected individuals and their families. Even among normally developing CYP, chronic sleep deprivation causes behavioural problems, impaired cognitive development and learning abilities, poor memory and attention problems, mood disorders and impaired school performances [3–5]. It also increases the risk of other health outcomes, such as obesity, cardiovascular, immunity, growth and metabolic consequences [6, 7]. It also significantly increases the stress level and impact the wellbeing of other family members and impair family cohesion [8]. Sleep disorders therefore further aggravate and exacerbate both internalising and externalising behaviours, emotional wellbeing and daily functioning of CYP with NDEBID. Appropriate management of sleep disorders ameliorate the short-term health and emotional consequences, optimization of daily functioning, family cohesion and prevention of psychiatric pathology in later adulthood [4, 9].

This chapter provides a brief summary of the extant literature on various important aspects of sleep physiology, aetiology, classification and prevalence of sleep disorders among CYP with NDEBIDs. It outlines various strategies for the management of sleep disorders, including behavioural non-pharmacological strategies and pharmacotherapy. Practical tips for clinicians managing CYP with co-morbid NDEBID and sleep disorders are outlined in an easy-to read flow chart, including sections on assessment, investigations, care plan formulation and follow-up.

## 2. What are neurodevelopmental (and related neurodisability), emotional, behavioural, intellectual and disorders (NDEBID)?

NDEBID is the umbrella terminology used in this chapter to refer to common childhood developmental disorders including several related conditions such as Attention Deficit/Hyperactivity Disorder (ADHD), Autism Spectrum Disorder (ASD), Cerebral palsy (CP), Epilepsy and Learning (Intellectual) disorders. Childhood NDEBID such as ADHD, tic disorder/Tourettes syndrome, developmental delay, development coordination disorder.

These conditions constitute a group of congenital or acquired long-term conditions that are attributed to disturbance of the brain and or neuromuscular system and create functional limitations in sensory, motor, speech, language, cognition or behaviour [10, 11]. They often co-occur together and co-morbidities are the rule rather than exceptions. Prevalence of up to 15% for NDEBID have been reported in developed countries, based on varying methodologies and definitions [12, 13]. They are best managed by specialist Paediatricians or Psychiatrists working within integrated teams involving other allied healthcare professionals, education, social care and voluntary sectors [14–16].

## 3. Sleep physiology in NDEBID

### 3.1 Definition and normal physiology

Sleep is a reversible state of reduced awareness of and responsiveness to the environment. There are two main phases of sleep: Rapid Eye Movement (REM) and

Non-REM [17]. Rapid eye movement (REM) sleep is prominent in early infancy, possibly explaining in part why sleep seems to be fragile at this age. Deep NREM sleep is particularly prominent in early childhood, and this is one of the reasons why arousal disorders (such as sleep walking) occur mainly at this stage [18].

### 3.2 What are the benefits and ideal sleep duration for children and adolescents?

Sleep is essential for optimal growth, emotional and cognitive development CYP. A group of experts from the American Academy of Sleep Medicine and the National Sleep Foundation have published recommendations for the sleep duration required by different age groups of CYP to refresh and rejuvenate the body and mind (**Table 1**).

Chronic sleep deprivation is associated with attention, behaviour, and learning problems, increased risk of accidents, injuries, hypertension, obesity, diabetes, and depression, as well increased risk of self-harm, suicidal thoughts, and suicide attempts among teenagers [19]. CYP and their carers require regular encouragement and emphasis about the benefits of adequate sleep, including improved attention, behaviour, learning, memory, emotional regulation, quality of life, mental and physical health (**Table 2**). Parents can help their children by monitoring their sleep pattern and encouraging them to see professionals for help.

| Age of the child | Recommended | May be appropriate | Not recommended |
|---|---|---|---|
| Newborn 0 to 3 months | 14 to 17 h | 11–19 h | including daytime naps |
| Infants* 4 to 12 months | 12 to 16 h | 10–18 h | including daytime naps |
| Children 1 to 2 years | 11 to 14 h | 9–16 h | including daytime naps |
| Pre-schoolers (3–5 yr) | 10–13 h | 8–14 h | Less than 8 h or more than 14 h |
| School-aged children (6–12 yr) | 9–12 h | 7–13 h | Less than 7 h or more than 12 h |
| Teenagers (13–18 yr) | 8–10 h | 7–11 h | Less than 7 h or more than 11 h |

**Table 1.**
*Recommended sleep duration for each age group.*

| Positive effects of adequate and good quality sleep | Negative consequences of lack of adequate and good quality sleep |
|---|---|
| • Promotes growth<br>• Strengthens immunity<br>• Helps cell growth and body repair<br>• Consolidates memory (https://www.sleepscotland.org/support/gateway-to-good-sleep/whyis-sleep-important/).<br>• Promotes learning and cognitive development.<br>• Maintains physical health and emotional wellbeing | • Increased association with excess weight gain and obesity.<br>• Impairs immune function.<br>• Affects physical coordination.<br>• Affects ability to learn new information and problem solve.<br>• Affects mood and emotional regulation and increases risk of mental health problems e.g., mood or anxiety disorder, suicidal ideation |

**Table 2.**
*Benefits of adequate sleep and negative consequences of inadequate sleep.*

### 3.3 Aetiology and pathogenesis of sleep disorders in NDEBID

The aetiology of sleep disorders in children with NDEBID is multifactorial and could also be disease specific. These include are biologic, behavioural (including environmental) and psycho-medical factors [20]. There is limited high-quality data and clinical guidelines to help offer a consistent approach to diagnosis and management of sleep disorders among CYP with NDEBID and co-morbid sleep problems [21]. **Table 3** shows common causes and examples of sleep disorders.

The most common sleep disorders among CYP include chronic sleep deprivation, delayed sleep phase disorder (especially among teenagers), difficulty falling asleep or maintaining sleep, and early morning [9, 22].

### 3.4 Classification of sleep disorders

Several terminologies and sometimes conflicting definitions of sleep disorders have been published, in terms of age, frequency, severity, and duration of symptoms. We refer to the definitions in both the 5th edition of Diagnostic and Statistical Manual of Mental Disorders (DSM-5) [18] and the 3rd edition of the International Classification of Sleep disorders (ICSD-3) [23] as reference standards in this chapter. Paediatric insomnia has been defined as "repeated difficulty with sleep initiation, duration, consolidation, or quality that occurs despite age-appropriate time and opportunity for

| | **Toddler/preschool (2–5 years)** | **School-aged (6–12 years)** | **Adolescent (13–1 8 years)** |
|---|---|---|---|
| 1. Bedtime | Does your child have any problems going to bed? Falling asleep | Does your child have any problems at bedtime? (P) Do you have any problems? (C) | Do you have any problems falling asleep at bedtime? (C) |
| 2. Excessive daytime sleepiness | Does your child seem overtired or sleep a lot during the day? Does she still take naps? | Does your child have difficulty waking in the morning, seem sleepy during the day or take naps? (P) Do you feel tired a lot? (C) | Do you feel sleepy a lot during the day? In school? While driving? (C) |
| 3. Awakenings during the night | Does your child wake up a lot at night? | Does your child seem to wake up a lot at night? Any sleepwalking or nightmares? (P) Do you wake up a lot at night? Have trouble getting back to sleep? (C) | Do you wake up a lot at night? Have trouble getting back to sleep? (C) |
| 4. Regularity and duration of sleep | Does your child have a regular bedtime and wake time? What are they? | What time does your child go to bed and get up on school days? Weekends? Do you think he/she is getting enough sleep (P) | What time do you usually go to bed on school nights? Weekends? How much sleep do you usually get? (C) |
| 5. Snoring | Does your child snore a lot or have difficulty breathing at night? | Does your child have loud or nightly snoring or any breathing difficulties | Does your teenager snore loudly or nightly? (P) |

*(P) Parent-directed question (C) Child-directed question. Source: Mindell JA, Owens JA. A Clinical Guide to Paediatric Sleep (Diagnosis and Management of Sleep Problems), Lippincott Williams & Wilkins 2003.*
**[B = bedtime problems; E = excessive daytime sleepiness; A = awakenings during the night; R = regularity and duration of sleep; S = Snoring].*

**Table 3.**
*Outline of 'BEARS'* screening questions.*

sleep and results in daytime functional impairment for the child and/or family" [6]. **Table 4** refers to a slightly modified ICSD-3 classification of sleep disorders.

### 3.5 Prevalence of sleep disorders in NDEBID

The commonest NDEBID mostly associated with sleep disorders include Autism spectrum disorder (ASD), Attention deficit hyperactivity disorder (ADHD) and Learning disabilities. Sleep disturbance is reported to be the second most common co-morbidity in children with ASD, with estimated prevalence between 33 and 81% [22, 24]. They often experience coexisting emotional problems such as anxiety or depression and epilepsy [25–27].

Common effects of sleep disturbances in CYP with ASD include increased severity of autism symptoms, challenging daytime behaviour such as physical aggression, emotional disturbances such as irritability, inattention, and hyperactivity [24, 28]. Several factors that may account for sleep disturbances associated with autism include alterations in neurotransmitter release, such as serotonin and melatonin, impaired

| Category | Description | Conditions and causes, some examples |
|---|---|---|
| Insomnias | Inability to fall asleep or stay asleep | Environmental: Poor sleep hygiene, bedroom noise, bright light.<br>Behavioural insomnia of childhood (sleep onset/limit setting/combined).<br>Psychiatric, trauma and substance misuse: Anxiety, depression, OCD, PTSD, abuse or neglect, bullying, drug and substance misuse.<br>Medical: Pain (headaches, ear ot toothaches, joint pains), lung problems (asthma, cystic fibrosis), skin (eczema, allergies), gastric reflux, neuromuscular, obesity, medication side effects. |
| Sleep related breathing disorders | Breathing difficulties during sleep | Obstructive sleep apnoea (including obesity, tonsil hypertrophy, facial dysmorphism, nasal septal deviation, craniofacial abnormalities, hypotonia, chronic rhinitis)<br>Central sleep apnoea |
| Central disorders of hypersomnolence | Excessively sleepy | Narcolepsy |
| Circadian rhythm sleep–wake disorders | Sleep times are out of alignment | Delayed sleep phase syndrome<br>Jet lag |
| Parasomnias | Unwanted events or experiences that occur at the time of falling asleep, sleeping or waking up | During NREM sleep: Confusional arousals, Sleep terrors, Sleepwalking<br>During REM sleep: Nightmares<br>Others: Enuresis or constipation |
| Sleep related movement disorders | Unusual body movements during sleep | Bruxism<br>Restless legs syndrome<br>Periodic limb movement disorder<br>Rhythmic movement disorder (head banging, body rocking) |

**Table 4.**
*ICSD-3 classification of common sleep disorders.*

sensory sensitization, behavioural insomnia syndromes, delayed sleep phase syndrome, abnormal rapid eye movement sleep, decreased time in bed, increased proportion of stage 1 sleep [25, 26].

Up to 70% of CYP with ADHD also have significant sleep problems including behavioural insomnia (limit-setting disorder), bedtime resistance, latency of sleep onset, dim light melatonin onset delay, decreased duration of sleep, increased number of overnight awakenings, and daytime somnolence sleep-disordered breathing, and restless legs syndrome/periodic limb movement disorder [29]. Their sleep disturbances may also be due to side-effects of ADHD medications [30]. Sleep problems among ADHD CYP can be transient and variable over time in up to 60% but can be more persistent in another 10% of the population [31]. Sleep problems can present with increasing severity of ADHD symptoms, poorer child quality of life (QoL), daily functioning and caregiver mental health, poor school performance and attendance [32]. It is important to emphasise that sleep disorders are identified before diagnosing ADHD, since disordered sleep can manifest with symptoms that mimic ADHD such as inattention, problematic behaviour, and poor emotional regulation [30].

## 4. Management of sleep disorders in CYP with NDEBID

### 4.1 Published clinical guidelines

There is limited global evidence-based clinical guidelines available to practitioners managing CYP with NDEBID [21]. Some professional bodies have produced multidisciplinary national consensus statements for the use of their members [7]. The American Academy of Neurology has also recently published treatment guidelines specifically addressing individuals with autism spectrum disorder [33]. The authors have published a proposed evidence-based flow chart practice guidance for managing sleep problems among CYP with NDEBID [34].

### 4.2 Clinical assessment

Clinical assessment with detailed medical, social, family, academic and lifestyle history including sleeping pattern and physical examinations during routine health encounters with CYP by all health practitioners should be undertaken as a standard procedure due to high prevalence of sleep problems in this population, especially among those with any NDEBID conditions [35, 36]. The diagnosis of sleep disorders in CYP is essentially clinical and should include information provided by the parents/caregivers and the older children and young people [7].

Sleep history should include the sleep/wake schedule, sleeping environment and bedtime routines, abnormal movements or behaviour during sleep, and lifestyle effects of sleep deprivation, daytime sleepiness, sleep onset latency and nighttime interruptions (**Box 1**) [2, 37].

Validated sleep questionnaires such as BEARS screening Assessment (see **Table 3**) and Children's Sleep Habit Questionnaire (CSHQ) are useful adjuncts to clinical assessment. The goal of detailed clinical assessment should be identification of a specified sleep disorder or of potential differential medical or anatomical diagnosis (**Table 4**). Detailed history about current medical conditions and medications should be recorded to determine possible effects on the sleep cycle (**Table 5**). Some co-existing medical conditions that may disturb sleep include Asthma, Eczema,

- Bedtime routines, nature of sleep environment, bedroom sharing and exposure to electronic gadgets
- Sleeping pattern including onset latency, nighttime awakening, abnormal movements or behaviour, night terrors and other parasomnias
- Levels of activity and exercise during the day
- Other physical, emotional or neurodevelopmental comorbidities including ADHD
- Physical illness or discomfort (for example, reflux, ear or toothache, bedwetting, constipation or eczema)
- Effects of any medications used and emotional state
- Any other factors affecting sleep, such as emotional relationships, challenging behaviours, school problems
- Impact of the sleep problems on parents or carers, other family members, school performances and other social functioning
- Family sleep patterns, parental expectations and cultural factors
- Clinical examination to exclude enlarged tonsils, facial dysmorphism, neurocutaneous markers etc.

**Box 1.**
*Components of detailed sleep assessment history.*

| Sleep-disturbance | Sleep-promoting |
|---|---|
| • Cholinergics .g. Methacholine, Carbachol, Pilocarpine and Pyridostigmine | • Anticholinergics e.g. Dicyclomine, Ipratropium, Hyoscine, Glycopyrrolate and Trihexyphenidyl |
| • Dopamine agonists e.g. pergolide and bromocriptine | • Dopamine antagonists e.g. Metoclopramide, Haloperidol, Melatonin and Risperidone |
| • Serotonin agonists e.g. Sumatriptan, Fluoxetine and Fenfluramine | • Serotonin Antagonists e.g. Cyproheptadine, Pizotifen and Mirtazapine |
| • Histamine agonists e.g. Methylhistamine, Cipralisant | • Antihistamines e.g. Chlorphenamine, Ranitidine, Cetrizine, Pizotifen and Olanzapine |
| • Adenosine antagonist e.g. Caffeine | • GABA agonists e.g. Baclofen and Benzodiazepines |

**Table 5.**
*Some medications that can influence the sleep cycle.*

Gastroesophageal reflux, Epilepsy, Chronic pain and Rheumatological conditions, and emotional problems like Anxiety, Depression and Mood disorders.

It should be noted that rare conditions like Narcolepsy and nocturnal Epilepsy are more commonly experienced co-morbidities among CYP with NDEBID [38].

### 4.3 Investigations

Baseline investigations required for formulation of a management plan include a 2-week sleep diary and actigraphy [9]. Actigraphy is a technical device used for monitoring body motion, sleep and wake patterns in individuals, that can be carried out in their home environment. It can measure sleep parameters such as total sleep time (TST), sleep efficiency, wake after sleep onset, and sleep onset latency (SOL), help to determine sleep patterns and document response to treatment in the patient's normal sleep [7].

Polysomnography (PSG) is a more comprehensive sleep study involving recording of sleep and other related physiological parameters from multiple electronic sensors, often combined with video recordings, carried out in specialist centres. PSG is particularly useful for diagnosis of sleep-related breathing disorder, atypical parasomnia, Periodic Limb movement disorder (PLMD), clinically unconfirmed Restless leg syndrome (RLS) or nocturnal seizures [39].

### 4.4 Common differential diagnosis and treatments

Detailed assessment should lead to formulation of a sleep disorder diagnosis or consideration of potential differential diagnosis including as follows:

#### *4.4.1 RLS and PLMD*

Common causes of childhood onset RLS include familial predisposition and systemic iron deficiency. Treatment options include iron supplementation and Gabapentin (researched mainly in adults). PLMD is a sleep disorder that is characterised by periodic and repetitive movements of legs and less often arms during sleep. Restless sleep disorder in childhood is a recently proposed entity, characterised by night-time restlessness, daytime sleepiness, and often iron deficiency, despite not meeting the diagnostic criteria for RLS or PLMD [17]. There is inconclusive research evidence for use of iron therapy, Dopamine agonists and anticonvulsants for RLS and PLMD in children [36].

#### *4.4.2 Parasomnias*

Parasomnias are undesirable physical activities predominantly associated with sleep. They are classified according to the dominant sleep phase during which they occur: rapid Eye Movement (REM), Non-REM and Non-specific. REM parasomnias include sleep paralysis, hallucinations and REM behaviour disorder. Non-REM parasomnias include confusional arousals (often triggered by sleep apnoea, RLS, or acid reflux), sleep walk and night terrors. Parasomnias often respond to reassurance and safety measures, with use of pharmacotherapy with benzodiazepines reserved for severe, potentially dangerous cases, and administered by sleep specialists [40].

#### *4.4.3 Obstructive sleep apnoea*

Obstructive sleep apnoea (OSA) is often caused by physical phenomenon such as adeno-tonsillar hypertrophy, cranio-facial anomalies, and obesity. The prevalence among CYP is estimated to be 2 percent and it is a common indication for urgent of children referral to the ENT surgeons [41].

#### *4.4.4 Delayed sleep phase syndrome (DSPS)*

Delayed Sleep Phase Syndrome (DSPS) is commonly diagnosed among male adolescents and associated with normal sleep pattern which is delayed by more than

*DOI: http://dx.doi.org/10.5772/intechopen.112031*

2 hours relative to socially acceptable conventional sleep times. It can be treated with chronotherapy, light therapy and potentially melatonin as long as the patient is motivated [42].

## 5. Comprehensive management of sleep disorders among CYP with NDEBID

A comprehensive clinical assessment should lead to the formulation of a sleep plan with graduated behavioural and pharmacological therapy and specialist referrals where indicated. The plan needs to be reviewed at regular intervals until a desirable sleep pattern has been achieved. A flow chart of recommended practice guidance is outlined in **Figure 1**.

### 5.1 Non-pharmacological/behavioural strategies

There is ample published evidence to recommend behavioural interventions as the first line treatment of sleep disorders, including practice of sleep hygiene, parent and care-giver education and training and behavioural interventions alternative therapies (such as massage therapy, aromatherapy, nutrients and multivitamin or iron supplementation) and Cognitive Behaviour Therapy (CBT) for older children and adolescents [9, 21, 26, 43].

#### *5.1.1 Behavioural strategies*

There is sufficient evidence to support the short- to medium-term effectiveness of cognitive-behavioural strategies based on learning principles, for the management of paediatric insomnia [7, 44]. The most popular behavioural interventions are different

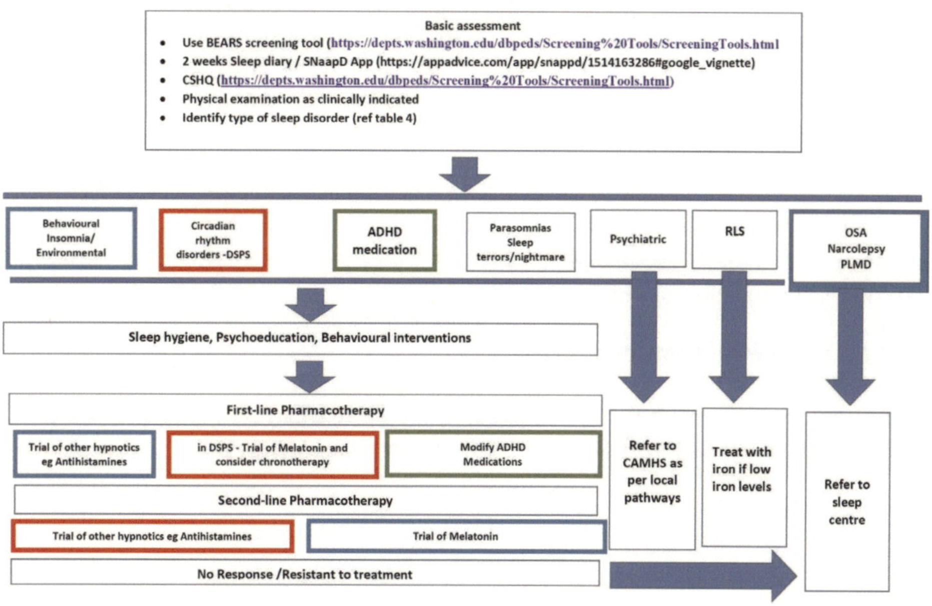


**Figure 1.**
*Recommended flow chart for sleep management guidance based on the published evidence.*

types of extinction: either complete (total removal of reinforcement to reduce a behaviour) or various degrees of graduated measures (including bedtime fading/positive routines and stimulus control techniques) and scheduled awakenings). The definitions and practical tips of cognitive behaviour strategies are listed in the **Table 6**.

#### *5.1.2 Parent-training and psychoeducation*

Psychoeducation is the process of empowering CYP and their carers by providing them with practical information regarding their sleep problems, with a systematic, structured and didactic approach [45, 46]. This enhanced understanding of their condition enables them to implement self-management strategies and effective partnership with professionals and improved compliance with prescribed treatment, resulting in more desirable outcomes. **Table 7** presents a list of some useful resources for parents and young people with sleep problems.

#### *5.1.3 Good sleep hygiene*

"Sleep hygiene" refers to healthy sleep habits and practical strategies that promote optimal sleeping patterns. They typically involve modifiable daytime, bedtime, and night-time practices such as diet, exercises and sleeping environment, with insufficient evidence to be recommended as stand-alone therapy [9, 37, 47]. Practical examples include use of reward charts, objects of reference such as applying parents pyjamas or perfume on teddy bear, pink or white noise (or music), night or daytime indicators such as Glo-clock or side lamps (**Box 1**).

#### *5.1.4 Cognitive behaviour therapy (CBT)*

CBT is a common psychological treatment that helps to modify negative thoughts and behaviours through structured conversation between the professional and the patient. There is scientific evidence that supports cognitive-behavioural treatment as the most effective intervention in the management of sleep disorders, especially for older adolescents and young people [7, 48].

#### *5.1.5 Neurofeedback*

Sensori-Motor Rhythm (SMR) and Slow-Cortical Potential (SCP) neurofeedback have been identified to produce some beneficial effects in improving sleep onset latency, especially among CYP with ADHD [49].

### 5.2 Pharmacological treatment

Pharmacotherapy is often considered as second line treatment after cognitive-behavioural strategies alone have not been effective.

#### *5.2.1 Melatonin*

Melatonin is a natural hormone produced by the pineal gland in the brain. It controls the body's circadian cycles which corresponds to the ambient 24 hour light–dark period, for such as sleep/wake rhythms, blood pressure, body temperature and metabolism [50]. The main effects of administered Melatonin include chronobiology

| Bedtime settling problems | | | | Night-time waking | | DSPS |
|---|---|---|---|---|---|---|
| **Extinction (Crying out)** | **Graduated extinction (Controlled crying)** | **Bedtime fading** | **Graded withdrawal** | **Robotic parent return** | **Scheduled awakening** | **Chronotherapy** |
| Parents need to ignore the child's crying for the child to self-soothe | This helps to take the 'flight' out of bedtime | Modified as some parents find this strategy less stressful. | Parent gradually withdraws from the child's bedroom to enable the child to fall asleep independently. | Parents need to avoid communication and interaction with the child when he/she wakes up at night, crying out loudly or calling out | This helps if the child wakes up frequently at the same time each night and cannot settle to sleep | This helps to reset the biological clock |
| Keep the regular bedtime<br>Completely Ignore the child's cries and calls | Keep the regular bedtime<br>Ignore the child's cries and calls for specific periods e.g., 3 minutes | Keep a sleep diary for 2 weeks to choose the new bedtime<br>Initially the child needs to stay up later, until their natural sleep time<br>Gradually move the bedtime earlier<br>Success within a few weeks | The child relies on the presence of parent to sleep<br>No change to bedtime needed<br>Withdraw from the child's bedroom gradually<br>Use with 'Robotic parent return' strategy<br>Success usually within 2 weeks | Do not carry or cuddle the child.<br>There should be no eye contact<br>Use magic phrase such as 'Time for sleep' but no other verbal communication<br>The child learns bedtime means sleep<br>Reward the child for better night's sleep and have lots of interaction with the child during daytime | Wake the child 15 to 30 minutes before the usual wake time<br>Use with 'Robotic parent return' strategy<br>Success within 2 weeks | Keep a sleep diary for 2 weeks to find out the bedtime and wake-up time<br>The adolescent needs to stay up 3 hours later and get up 3 hours later than the established sleep/wake schedule<br>Avoid naps |

*Source: "Sleep problems in children and young people: A simple teaching aid", a flip chart written by Dr. CR Yemula, Andrea Roberts and edited by professor Besag).*

**Table 6.**
*Behavioural interventions to improve sleep in children with chronic insomnia.*

| Users | Resources | Free access | Website links |
|---|---|---|---|
| Parents and carers | CEREBRA-Sleep Advice service | Yes | https://cerebra.org.uk/get-advice-support/sleep-advice-service/ |
| | Sleep for better day ahead leaflet | Yes | https://www.qvh.nhs.uk/wp-content/uploads/2020/08/Sleep-for-a-better-day-ahead- 0127.pdf |
| | Sleep hygiene in children and young people: Information for families-leaflet | Yes | https://media.gosh.nhs.uk/documents/Sleep_hygiene_F1851_FINAL_Jun20.pdf |
| | Encouraging good sleep habits in children with learning disabilities-leaflet | Yes | https://www.oxfordhealth.nhs.uk/wp-content/uploads/2014/05/Good-sleep-habits-forchildren-with-Learning-Difficulties.pdf |
| | Sleep problems and sleep disorders in school aged children | Yes | https://www.sleephealthfoundation.org.au/sleep-problemsand-sleep-disorders-inschool-aged-children.html |
| | Further useful facts sheets and resources-website | Yes | https://www.sleephealthfoundation.org.au/fact-sheets.html |
| | Other websites | Yes | https://www.nhs.uk/live-well/sleep-and-tiredness/healthy-sleep-tips-for-children/; https://www.sleepscotland.org/ |
| Adolescents | How to sleep well and stay healthy-A guide for teenagers. This is an interactive apple book with animations, sounds and external links to useful educational video clips | Yes | https://books.apple.com/gb/book/how-to-sleep-well-and-stay-healthy-a-guide-forteenagers/id1397176909 It is available for iPad, iPhone and MAC book. |
| | How to sleep well -Teen sleep guide This is an interactive pdf guide | Yes | https://www.cambscommunityservices.nhs.uk/docs/default-source/bedfordshire-childrens-services/beds—books/teen-sleep-guide-14-sep-2022.pdf?sfvrsn=2 |
| | Sleep tips for teenagers | Yes | https://www.nhs.uk/live-well/sleep-and-tiredness/sleep-tips-for-teenagers/ |
| Children | Sleep poster: Interactive pdf for children and parents/carers | Yes | https://www.cambscommunityservices.nhs.uk/docs/default-source/Luton—NDDWebpages/Sleep/sleep-poster76ddec06f4f66239b188ff0000d24525.pdf?sfvrsn = 2 |
| | I see the animals sleeping: A bedtime story-an app | Free on Google play, App store and Kindle store | http://school.sleepeducation.com/childrensapps.aspx |
| | The animal sleep: A bedtime book for biomes-an app | | http://school.sleepeducation.com/childrensapps.aspx; https://www.youtube.com/watch?v=zLQ3bkn8Gu8 |

**Table 7.**
*Some useful resources for parents and adolescents.*

(circadian phase-shifting) and hypnosis (sleep-promotion). Melatonin also has some immune modulating properties and should be avoided in individuals with compromised immune functioning [51].

There is ample published evidence to support the use of melatonin in treating CYP with NDEBID. The reported benefits of moderate doses of melatonin (up to 6 mg) include reduced sleep onset latency and number of awakenings/night, and increase in total hours of sleep/night [52–54], but it has no significant benefit in reducing the number of awakenings per night [54], and has limited effect on Child behaviour and family functioning [55]. Melatonin is more likely going to be effective for children who are sleeping less than 6 hours at night [56]. However, there is a paucity of evidence on managing sleep disturbances in CYP with NDEBID specifically [57].

Most slow-release melatonin formulations (mainly Circadin) are licenced for adults with primary insomnia, but are widely used "off-label" to treat sleep disorders among CYP of all ages [58]. The European Medicines Agency has recently licenced a melatonin brand (Slenyto) for CYP with Autism and Smith Magenis syndrome [59]. The U.S. Food and Drug Administration recognises Melatonin as a supplement which therefore does has not require its *approval*. Melatonin is generally considered to be safe for short-term management of sleep disorders among CYP, but its long-term safety have not been extensively studied [60]. CYP on melatonin require regular re-evaluation to ensure the treatment is terminated as soon as it is no longer required [50].

The effectiveness of melatonin can often diminish overt time, due to decreased the CYP1A2 liver enzyme activity, either genetically determined or due to the effect of other medications [61]. In patients with loss of response to melatonin, a period of melatonin clearance for up to 3 weeks and a considerable dose reduction has been advised [20].

#### *5.2.2 Antihistamines (alimemazine, promethazine, diphenhydramine, hydroxyzine)*

Antihistamines constitute the most popular prescribed agents for managing sleep problems among CYP with sleep problems, despite limited research evidence to support their efficacy. Clinicians should be aware that some sedative antihistamines, such as hydroxyzine or diphenhydramine can present with paradoxical agitations in children, and their effects on sleep latency duration is very minimal [54].

#### *5.2.3 Alpha 2 adrenergic agonists (clonidine and Guanfacine)*

Clonidine and Guanfacine are examples of alpha-2-adrenergic receptor agonist, whose mechanism of action for sedation remains elusive. They are commonly prescribed for CYP with co-morbid ADHD and associated sleep disorders, but the research evidence to support their effectiveness is very scanty [49, 62]. In a USA National survey, alpha agonists were the most commonly prescribed insomnia medication for children with ADHD (81%) [63].

#### *5.2.4 Z-drugs (zopiclone, eszopiclone, zaleplon and zolpidem)*

Z-drugs are approved and commonly prescribed for transient sleep disorders in adults. Only few studies have been carried out regarding effectiveness among CYP, with contrasting results, and report of increased adverse effects compared to melatonin [37, 55].

### *5.2.5 Benzodiazepines (like clonazepam and Flurazepam)*

Benzodiazepines are sedative medications which are not routinely recommended for treatment of sleep disorders in children, except for limited periods to alleviate co-morbid daytime anxiety [37]. Clonazepam has been advocated for treatment of severe parasomnia/night terrors under specialist supervision [47].

### *5.2.6 Selective serotonin reuptake inhibitors (SSRIs) and tricyclic antidepressants*

Use of selective serotonin reuptake inhibitors (SSRIs) such as Sertraline may be considered for disabling bedtime anxiety. Tricyclic antidepressants, used in adults with insomnia, are not approved for CYP due to their poor safety profile [47]. While Trazodone and mirtazapine have potential benefits, they require further evidence for routine prescription for children with NDEBID [37]. Trazodone may be effective in managing sleep disorders among children with Angelman syndrome with specialist advice from a tertiary sleep centre [47].

## 6. Alternative therapies

There is a plethora of herbal and other over-the-counter formulations that have traditional been used for self-management of sleep disturbances, based on anecdotal assumptions. These include Valerian, Lavender, Chamomile and Kava products [7].

## 7. Combined treatment modalities

Only limited studies have assessed the efficacy combining behavioural and pharmacological therapies. The combination of controlled-release melatonin over 12 weeks and four sessions of cognitive-behavioural therapy among a group of ASD Children aged 4–10 years, showed a trend to outperform other active treatment groups, with fewer dropouts and a greater proportion of treatment responders achieving clinically significant changes [64].

A similar small Canadian study among 27 ADHD children reported the effect size of the combined sleep hygiene and melatonin intervention from baseline to 90 days' posttrial was 1.7, compared to 0.6 on average for either sleep hygiene or melatonin alone. However, the decreased sleep latency and improved sleep had no demonstrable effect on ADHD symptoms [65].

## 8. Referrals to relevant specialist

Considering the limited resources and varied expertise in clinical practice, it is important for clinicians to have a low threshold to make an onward referral whenever a significant sleep disorder is suspected. The referral pathways/practice policies need to be agreed locally among all the major Clinicians and stakeholders [39].

Sleep disorders that often require further evaluation by a specialist include suspected OSA, PLMD, debilitating parasomnias and narcolepsy. Referrals should be made to a relevant specialist such as an ENT surgeon (in case of suspected OSA) or a

Respiratory physician/sleep centre for suspected severe parasomnias, PLMD or narcolepsy [17].

## 9. Conclusion

Children and young people with neurodevelopmental disorders experience higher prevalence of sleep difficulties and sleep disorders compared to the general population. In addition to other associated comorbidity, this can negatively affect their cognitive development, behaviour, physical and mental health. There is also significant negative impact on their peer- and family-relationships.

In view of the high prevalence of associated sleep problems, clinicians should screen for sleep disorders when assessing all children and adolescents with cognitive, behavioural, and emotional problems. It is important to undertake a comprehensive evaluation, including use of clinical tools such as BEARS questionnaire, Child Sleep Habit Questionnaire, a 2-week sleep diary, actigraphy and relevant physical examination, in order to identify the sleep pattern and diagnose and any underlying potential sleep disorders.

Due to the complex nature of underlying comorbidity, social, cognitive and psychological difficulties, it is often a frustrating journey for parents/carers to achieve a good quality of sleep for CYP with NDEBID. Initial steps in management involve providing parents/carers and CYP with user-friendly psychoeducation and sleep hygiene measures, taking into account the individual and family circumstances. Specific behavioural interventions where appropriate can be implemented as first line management for sleep disorders.

In CYP with NDEBID and insomnia, use of melatonin should be carefully considered only following an unsuccessful trial of sleep hygiene and behavioural measures, while persevering with the appropriate sleep hygiene measures. Referrals should be made to relevant specialist/sleep centre for further assessment and management of severe sleep disorders, including OSA, PLMD and narcolepsy.

## Conflict of interest

The authors declare no conflict of interest.

## Abbreviations

| | |
|---|---|
| ADHD | Attention Deficit/Hyperactivity Disorder |
| ASD | Autism Spectrum Disorder |
| CP | Cerebral palsy |
| Epilepsy and ID | Intellectual (Learning) disorders |
| NDD | Neurodevelopmental disorders |
| NDEBID | Neurodevelopmental (and related Neurodisability), Emotional, Behavioural, Intellectual and Disorders |
| CYP | Children and Young people |
| SOL | sleep-onset latency |
| SOI | sleep-onset insomnia |
| TST | total sleep time. |

## Author details

Michael O. Ogundele[1*], Chinnaiah Yemula[2] and Hani F. Ayyash[3,4,5,6]

1 Department of Community Paediatrics, Bridgewater Community Healthcare NHS Foundation Trust, Halton District, UK

2 Department of Community Paediatrics, Cambridgeshire Community Services NHS Trust, St Ives, Cambridgeshire

3 Essex Partnership University NHS Foundation Trust, Essex, United Kingdom

4 Children's Health Services, Southend-On-Sea, United Kingdom

5 British Paediatric Surveillance Unit, Royal College of Paediatrics and Child Health, London, United Kingdom

6 Child and Adolescent Psychiatry Surveillance System, Royal College of Psychiatrists, London, United Kingdom

*Address all correspondence to: m.ogundele@nhs.net

## References

[1] Vélez-Galarraga R, Guillén-Grima F, Crespo-Eguílaz N, Sánchez-Carpintero R. 'Prevalence of sleep disorders and their relationship with core symptoms of inattention and hyperactivity in children with attention-deficit/hyperactivity disorder'. European Journal of Paediatric Neurology, Nov. 2016;**20**(6):925-937. DOI: 10.1016/j.ejpn.2016.07.004

[2] Meltzer LJ, Crabtree VM. Pediatric Sleep Problems: A clinician's Guide to Behavioral Interventions. Washington, DC, US: American Psychological Association; 2015. pp. xv, 282. DOI: 10.1037/14645-000

[3] Calhoun SL, Fernandez-Mendoza J, Vgontzas AN, Mayes SD, Liao D, Bixler EO. Behavioral profiles associated with objective sleep duration in young children with insomnia symptoms. Journal of Abnormal Child Psychology. 2017;**45**(2):337-344. DOI: 10.1007/s10802-016-0166-4

[4] Licis A. Sleep disorders: Assessment and treatment in preschool-aged children. Child and Adolescent Psychiatric Clinics of North America. 2017;**26**(3):587-595. DOI: 10.1016/j.chc.2017.02.009

[5] Scammell TE. Overview of sleep: The neurologic processes of the sleep-wake cycle. The Journal of Clinical Psychiatry. 2015;**76**(5):e13. DOI: 10.4088/JCP.14046tx1c

[6] Meltzer LJ, Mindell JA. Systematic review and meta-analysis of behavioral interventions for pediatric insomnia. Journal of Pediatric Psychology. 2014;**39**(8):932-948. DOI: 10.1093/jpepsy/jsu041

[7] Pin Arboledas G et al. Insomnia in children and adolescents. A consensus document. Anales de Pediatría. 2017;**86**(3):165.e1-165.e11. DOI: 10.1016/j.anpede.2016.06.002

[8] Byars KC, Yeomans-Maldonado G, Noll JG. Parental functioning and pediatric sleep disturbance: An examination of factors associated with parenting stress in children clinically referred for evaluation of insomnia. Sleep Medicine. 2011;**12**(9):898-905. DOI: 10.1016/j.sleep.2011.05.002

[9] Shatkin JP, Pando M. Diagnosis and treatment of common sleep disorders in adolescence. Adolescent Psychiatry. 2015;**5**(3):146-163

[10] Ogundele MO, Morton M. Classification, prevalence and integrated care for neurodevelopmental and child mental health disorders: A brief overview for paediatricians. World Journal of Clinical Pediatrics. 2022;**11**(2):120-135. DOI: 10.5409/wjcp.v11.i2.120

[11] Gillberg C, Fernell E, Minnis H. Early symptomatic syndromes eliciting neurodevelopmental clinical examinations. Scientific World Journal. 2014;**2013**:710570. DOI: 10.1155/2013/710570

[12] Morris C, Janssens A, Tomlinson R, Williams J, Logan S. Towards a definition of neurodisability: A Delphi survey. Developmental Medicine and Child Neurology. 2013;**55**(12):1103-1108. DOI: 10.1111/dmcn.12218

[13] World health Organization (WHO) by Buka, I, 'Children and Neurodevelopmental Behavioural Intellectual Disorders (NDBID). WHO Training Package for the Health Sector.' WHO; 2011 [Online]. Available from: https://www.who.int/ceh/capacity/neurodevelopmental.pdf [Accessed: June 10, 2020].

[14] Ogundele MO. A profile of common neurodevelopmental disorders presenting in a Scottish community child health service –a one year audit (2016/ 2017). HR. 2018;**2**(1):1. DOI: 10.31058/j.hr.2018.21001

[15] Ogundele MO, Ayyash HF. Integrated Services for Children and Young People with neurodevelopmental and Co-morbid mental health disorders: Review of the evidence. Journal of Psychiatry & Mental Disorders. 2020; **5**(3):1027

[16] Ani C, Ayyash HF, Ogundele MO. Community paediatricians' experience of joint working with child and adolescent mental health services: Findings from a British national survey. BMJPO. 2022;**6**(1):e001381. DOI: 10.1136/bmjpo-2021-001381

[17] Licis A. Sleep-Wake Disorders in Childhood. Continuum (Minneap Minn). 2020;**26**(4):1034-1069. DOI: 10.1212/CON.0000000000000897

[18] American Psychiatric Association (APA). Diagnostic and Statistical Manual of Mental Disorders (DSM-5). Fifth ed. Washington, DC, USA: American Psychiatric Association; 2013. DOI: 10.1176/appi.books.9780890425596

[19] Paruthi S et al. Recommended amount of sleep for pediatric populations: A consensus statement of the American Academy of sleep medicine. Journal of Clinical Sleep Medicine. 2016;**12**(6):785-786. DOI: 10.5664/jcsm.5866

[20] Braam W, van Geijlswijk I, Keijzer H, Smits MG, Didden R, Curfs LMG. Loss of response to melatonin treatment is associated with slow melatonin metabolism. Journal of Intellectual Disability Research. 2010; **54**(6):547-555. DOI: 10.1111/j.1365-2788.2010.01283.x

[21] Blackmer AB, Feinstein JA. Management of Sleep Disorders in children with neurodevelopmental disorders: A review. Pharmacotherapy. 2016;**36**(1): 84-98. DOI: 10.1002/phar.1686

[22] Reed HE et al. Parent-based sleep education workshops in autism. Journal of Child Neurology. 2009;**24**(8): 936-945. DOI: 10.1177/0883073808331348

[23] 'International Classification of Sleep Disorders – Third Edition (ICSD-3) (Online)'. Available from: https://learn.aasm.org/Public/Catalog/Details.aspx?id=%2FgqQVDMQIT%2FEDy86PWgqgQ%3D%3D&returnurl=%2FUsers%2FUserOnlineCourse.aspx%3FLearningActivityID%3D%252fgqQVDMQIT%252fEDy86PWgqgQ%253d%253d [Accessed: February 7, 2021]

[24] Mannion A, Leader G. Sleep problems in autism Spectrum disorder: A literature review. Review Journal of Autism and Developmental Disorders. 2014;**1**(2):101-109. DOI: 10.1007/s40489-013-0009-y

[25] Devnani PA, Hegde AU. Autism and sleep disorders. Journal of Pediatric Neurosciences. 2015;**10**(4):304-307. DOI: 10.4103/1817-1745.174438

[26] Mazurek MO, Petroski GF. Sleep problems in children with autism spectrum disorder: Examining the contributions of sensory over-responsivity and anxiety. Sleep Medicine. 2015;**16**(2):270-279. DOI: 10.1016/j.sleep.2014.11.006

[27] Tsai M-H, Hsu J-F, Huang Y-S. Sleep problems in children with attention deficit/hyperactivity disorder: Current status of knowledge and appropriate

management. Current Psychiatry Reports. 2016;**18**(8):76. DOI: 10.1007/s11920-016-0711-4

[28] Mazurek MO, Sohl K. Sleep and behavioral problems in children with autism Spectrum disorder. Journal of Autism and Developmental Disorders. 2016;**46**(6):1906-1915. DOI: 10.1007/s10803-016-2723-7

[29] Ogundele MO. Management of sleep difficulties among a cohort of children with adhd in a scottish local authority. Archives of Disease in Childhood. 2018; **103**(Suppl. 1):A190-A191. DOI: 10.1136/archdischild-2018-rcpch.455

[30] Cortese S et al. Assessment and Management of Sleep Problems in youths with attention-deficit/hyperactivity disorder. Journal of the American Academy of Child and Adolescent Psychiatry. 2013;**52**:784-796. DOI: 10.1016/j.jaac.2013.06.001

[31] Lycett K, Mensah FK, Hiscock H, Sciberras E. A prospective study of sleep problems in children with ADHD. Sleep Medicine. 2014;**15**(11):1354-1361. DOI: 10.1016/j.sleep.2014.06.004

[32] Sciberras E, Fulton M, Efron D, Oberklaid F, Hiscock H. Managing sleep problems in school aged children with ADHD: A pilot randomised controlled trial. Sleep Medicine. 2011;**12**(9): 932-935. DOI: 10.1016/j.sleep.2011.02.006

[33] Williams Buckley A et al. Practice guideline: Treatment for insomnia and disrupted sleep behavior in children and adolescents with autism spectrum disorder: Report of the guideline development, dissemination, and implementation Subcommittee of the American Academy of neurology. Neurology. 2020;**94**(9):392-404. DOI: 10.1212/WNL.0000000000009033

[34] Ogundele MO, Yemula C. Management of sleep disorders among children and adolescents with neurodevelopmental disorders: A practical guide for clinicians - PMC. World Journal of Clinical Pediatrics. 2022;**11**(3):239-252. DOI: 10.5409/wjcp.v11.i3.239

[35] Ogundele MO. Behavioural and emotional disorders in childhood: A brief overview for paediatricians. World Journal of Clinical Pediatrics. 2018;**7**(1): 9-26. DOI: 10.5409/wjcp.v7.i1.9

[36] Esposito S et al. Pediatric sleep disturbances and treatment with melatonin. Journal of Translational Medicine. 2019;**17**(1):77. DOI: 10.1186/s12967-019-1835-1

[37] Bruni O, Angriman M, Melegari MG, Ferri R. Pharmacotherapeutic management of sleep disorders in children with neurodevelopmental disorders. Expert Opinion on Pharmacotherapy. 2019;**20**(18):2257-2271. DOI: 10.1080/14656566.2019.1674283

[38] Miano S, Esposito M, Foderaro G, Ramelli GP, Pezzoli V, Manconi M. Sleep-related disorders in children with attention-deficit hyperactivity disorder: Preliminary results of a full sleep assessment study. CNS Neuroscience & Therapeutics. 2016;**22**(11):906-914. DOI: 10.1111/cns.12573

[39] Silvestri R, Ipsiroglu OS. Behavioral sleep medicine—The need for harmonization of clinical best practice outcome measures in children and adolescents with intellectual or developmental disabilities and restless sleep. Frontiers in Psychiatry. 2022;**13**:1003019. DOI: 10.3389/fpsyt.2022.1003019

[40] Simon SL, Byars KC. Behavioral treatments for non-rapid eye movement

parasomnias in children. Current Sleep Medicine Reports. 2016;**2**(3): 152-157. DOI: 10.1007/s40675-016-0049-9

[41] Rosen GM, Morrissette S, Larson A, Stading P, Barnes TL. Does improvement of low serum ferritin improve symptoms of restless legs syndrome in a cohort of pediatric patients? Journal of Clinical Sleep Medicine. 2019;**15**(8):1149-1154. DOI: 10.5664/jcsm.7810

[42] Boivin DB. Treating delayed sleep-wake phase disorder in young adults - PubMed. Journal of Psychiatry & Neuroscience. 2017;**42**(5):E9-E10. DOI: 10.1503/jpn.160243

[43] Mindell JA et al. Pharmacologic Management of Insomnia in children and adolescents: Consensus statement. Pediatrics. 2006;**117**(6):e1223-e1232. DOI: 10.1542/peds.2005-1693

[44] Kotagal S. Treatment of dyssomnias and parasomnias in childhood. Current Treatment Options in Neurology. 2012; **14**(6):630-649. DOI: 10.1007/s11940-012-0199-0

[45] Dahl V et al. Psychoeducation interventions for parents and teachers of children and adolescents with ADHD: A systematic review of the literature. Journal of Developmental and Physical Disabilities. 2020;**32**(2):257-292. DOI: 10.1007/s10882-019-09691-3

[46] Sarkhel S, Singh OP, Arora M. Clinical practice guidelines for psychoeducation in psychiatric disorders general principles of psychoeducation-PMC. Indian Journal of Psychiatry. 2020;**62**(Suppl 2):S319-S323. DOI: 10.4103/psychiatry

[47] McDonald A, Joseph D. Paediatric neurodisability and sleep disorders: Clinical pathways and management strategies. BMJ Paediatrics Open. 2019; **3**(1):e000290. DOI: 10.1136/bmjpo-2018-000290

[48] Blake MJ, Sheeber LB, Youssef GJ, Raniti MB, Allen NB. Systematic review and meta-analysis of adolescent cognitive-behavioral sleep interventions. Clinical Child and Family Psychology Review. 2017;**20**(3):227-249. DOI: 10.1007/s10567-017-0234-5

[49] Arns M, Kenemans JL. Neurofeedback in ADHD and insomnia: Vigilance stabilization through sleep spindles and circadian networks. Neuroscience and Biobehavioral Reviews. 2014;**44**:183-194. DOI: 10.1016/j.neubiorev.2012.10.006

[50] Janjua I, Goldman RD. Sleep-related melatonin use in healthy children. Canadian Family Physician. 2016;**62**(4): 315-317

[51] Pelayo R, Yuen K. Pediatric sleep pharmacology. Child and Adolescent Psychiatric Clinics of North America. 2012;**21**(4):861-883. DOI: 10.1016/j.chc.2012.08.001

[52] Ayyash HF, Preece P, Morton R, Cortese S. Melatonin for sleep disturbance in children with neurodevelopmental disorders: Prospective observational naturalistic study. Expert Review of Neurotherapeutics. 2015;**15**(6): 711-717. DOI: 10.1586/14737175.2015.1041511

[53] Abdelgadir IS, Gordon MA, Akobeng AK. Melatonin for the management of sleep problems in children with neurodevelopmental disorders: A systematic review and meta-analysis. Archives of Disease in Childhood. 2018;**103**(12):1155-1162. DOI: 10.1136/archdischild-2017-314181

[54] McDonagh MS, Holmes R, Hsu F. Pharmacologic treatments for sleep disorders in children: A systematic review. Journal of Child Neurology. 2019;**34**(5):237-247. DOI: 10.1177/0883073818821030

[55] Gringras P et al. Melatonin for sleep problems in children with neurodevelopmental disorders: Randomised double masked placebo controlled trial. BMJ. 2012;**345**:e6664. DOI: 10.1136/bmj.e6664

[56] Appleton RE et al. The use of MElatonin in children with neurodevelopmental disorders and impaired sleep: A randomised, double-blind, placebo-controlled, parallel study (MENDS). Health Technology Assessment. 2012;**16**(40):i-239. DOI: 10.3310/hta16400

[57] Parker A et al. Oral melatonin for non-respiratory sleep disturbance in children with neurodisabilities: Systematic review and meta-analyses. Developmental Medicine and Child Neurology. 2019;**61**(8):880-890. DOI: 10.1111/dmcn.14157

[58] Chua HM, Hauet Richer N, Swedrowska M, Ingham S, Tomlin S, Forbes B. Dissolution of intact, divided and crushed Circadin tablets: Prolonged vs. immediate release of melatonin. Pharmaceutics. 2016;**8**(1):2. DOI: 10.3390/pharmaceutics8010002

[59] European Medicines Agency (EMA). Two New Paediatric-Use Marketing Authorisations Recommended by CHMP. London, UK: European Medicines Agency; 2018

[60] Schwichtenberg AJ, Malow BA. Melatonin treatment in children with developmental disabilities. Sleep Medicine Clinics. 2015;**10**(2):181-187. DOI: 10.1016/j.jsmc.2015.02.008

[61] Bruni O et al. Current role of melatonin in pediatric neurology: Clinical recommendations. European Journal of Paediatric Neurology. 2015;**19**(2):122-133. DOI: 10.1016/j.ejpn.2014.12.007

[62] Anand S, Tong H, Besag FMC, Chan EW, Cortese S, Wong ICK. Safety, tolerability and efficacy of drugs for treating Behavioural insomnia in children with attention-deficit/hyperactivity disorder: A systematic review with methodological quality assessment. Paediatric Drugs. 2017;**19**(3):235-250. DOI: 10.1007/s40272-017-0224-6

[63] Owens J et al. Future research directions in sleep and ADHD: Report of a consensus working group. Journal of Attention Disorders. 2013;**17**(7):550-564. DOI: 10.1177/1087054712457992

[64] Cortesi F, Giannotti F, Sebastiani T, Panunzi S, Valente D. Controlled-release melatonin, singly and combined with cognitive behavioural therapy, for persistent insomnia in children with autism spectrum disorders: A randomized placebo-controlled trial. Journal of Sleep Research. 2012;**21**(6):700-709. DOI: 10.1111/j.1365-2869.2012.01021.x

[65] Weiss MD, Wasdell MB, Bomben MM, Rea KJ, Freeman RD. Sleep hygiene and melatonin treatment for children and adolescents with ADHD and initial insomnia. Journal of the American Academy of Child and Adolescent Psychiatry. 2006;**45**(5):512-519. DOI: 10.1097/01 chi.0000205706.78818.ef

Chapter 5

# Common Sleep Problems and Management in Older Adults

*Pak Wing Cheng and Yiu Pan Wong*

## Abstract

Sleep problems are common among the elderly due to physiological changes and comorbid psychiatric and medical conditions. Sleep architecture changes with age. However, sleep disturbances among older adults should not be seen barely as a result of ageing. Depression and anxiety are important differential diagnoses for elderly patients complaining of sleep disturbance. Dementia and delirium are also common causes of sleep disturbances among older people. Elderly people often carry several medical comorbidities. These medical conditions can both lead to and be exacerbated by sleep problems. Given the frailty, multimorbidity and vulnerability of some of the elderly, the management of sleep problems requires additional considerations compared with younger adult patients. Behavioural modifications and drugs of choice will be discussed.

**Keywords:** elderly, sleep disturbance, insomnia, geriatric psychiatry, insomnia management

## 1. Introduction

Sleep problems are common in the elderly population. A recent meta-analysis study suggested that the prevalence of pooled sleep disturbance was up to 35.9% in older Chinese adults [1]. Another study in Italy suggested that insomnia was observed in 44.2% of subjects aged 65 or above [2]. While causes of sleep disturbance among the elderly are multi-folded, it is clear that female gender, depressed mood and physical illnesses are general risk factors for sleep disturbance in the geriatric population [3]. Other less robust risk factors in this age group identified by different studies include low physical activity level, low economic status, loneliness and perceived stress [3]. Mild cognitive impairment, long-term use of sedative drugs and high inflammatory markers are also possible predicting sleep disturbance factors [3]. While psychical health issues can affect sleep, poor sleep, in turn, can exacerbate mood and medical problems, causing a vicious cycle. For example, Eguchi et al. [4] demonstrated in their study that short sleep duration is an independent predictor of stroke among the elderly with hypertension. It was also suggested that difficulties in initiating sleep and maintaining sleep in people aged 75 or above were associated with an increased risk of falls, which is a particular worry for elderly people [5]. Poor sleep is closely related to cognitive decline and the mental health of elderly people. However, these problems are often unaware by medical professionals or not optimally and timely managed. The following paragraphs aim to present a general picture of sleep problems in senior groups.

## 2. Sleep cycle and pattern of the elderly

Studies have shown that amount of sleep and sleep architecture change with age. On the one hand, total sleep time, deep slow-wave sleep and sleep efficiency (the ratio of total sleep time to time in bed) decrease with age [6]. A more recent study done by Schwarz et al. [7] on elderly women further suggests that ageing was associated with lower fast spindle and K-complex density in N2. On the other hand, the duration of light sleep increases with age, with elderly people being more easily awakened by external stimuli and resulting in sleep fragmentation [8, 9]. In a study done by Ohayon and Vecchierini [10], the median night-time sleep duration of elderly people aged 60 or above was about 7 hours, with no significant difference found among different sub-age groups of these elderly people. The authors suggested that a short total sleep time was associated with obesity, poor health and cognitive impairment [10]. Therefore, short sleep time and insomnia among the elderly population should not be attributed to ageing alone [10–12].

Advanced sleep phase syndrome is another key feature of elderly sleep patterns [9, 13]. Elderly people tend to go to sleep and wake up earlier compared with young adults. Biologically, this can be a result of the decrease in the suprachiasmatic nucleus(SCN) volume and cell count and a decrease in melatonin secretion [13, 14]. Various other physiological malfunction processes at the cellular and systematic levels also contribute to circadian desynchrony and alternation of sleep patterns among elder people [13]. Psychosocially, advanced sleep phase syndrome can also result from lifestyle changes after retirement and subsequently reduced light exposure [8, 13]. With a generally more sedentary and less social lifestyle, there is little drive for older adults with advanced sleep phase syndrome to reschedule their bedtime [8].

## 3. Insomnia and mood disorders among the elderly

### 3.1 Insomnia

Insomnia is the predominant sleep problem found among the elderly population. While there are no well-recognised diagnostic criteria or classification systems dedicated to insomnia disorder in the senior age group, a general framework for insomnia can be used in the encounter with elderly patients. According to DSM-5, insomnia disorder refers to dissatisfaction with the quality and quantity of sleep that cause distress or impairment in daily function [15]. To fulfil the diagnostic criteria of insomnia disorder, one has to experience sleep difficulty despite sufficient chances to sleep, and the sleep difficulty should last for at least three days a week [15]. Sleep difficulty could arise from difficulties in falling asleep (sleep initiation), frequent awakening and difficulty in returning to sleep (sleep maintenance) or early-morning awakening (late insomnia) [15]. Sleep fragmentation is common in the elderly population, especially those with dementia. Demented patients, as mentioned below, are also subject to early morning awakening.

Insomnia disorder can be classified according to its chronicity and aetiology. According to the International Classification of Sleep Disorders (ICSD)-Third

Edition, insomnia is considered chronic for over three months [16]. ICSD classifies the aetiology of insomnia into primary and comorbid [16]. Similarly, DSM-5 includes specifiers of insomnia according to the comorbid conditions, i.e. with non-sleep disorder mental comorbidity, with other medical comorbidity and other sleep disorders [15]. Elderly patients are subject to multiple comorbidities and polypharmacy. Insomnia is a common result of these chronic conditions. Therefore, the diagnosis of chronic insomnia is better reserved for patients for whom insomnia is especially prominent, unexpectedly prolonged and is one of the foci of treatment plans [16]. Pharmacological treatments for chronic insomnia in the elderly should be prescribed with caution in view of the possible serious side effects of certain drugs among elderly patients (see below).

As with other psychiatric conditions, the causation of insomnia can be understood in terms of biological mechanisms and psychosocial aspects. The two-process model of sleep–wake regulation depicts the roles of melatonin and adenosine, which regulate circadian rhythm regulation and sleep–wake homeostasis, respectively [17]. Dysregulation of the circadian rhythm can lead to difficulty in sleep initiation and early morning awakening, while dysregulation of sleep–wake homeostasis may lead to sleep initiation and maintenance difficulties [17]. Cajochen et al. [18] suggested that age-related changes in sleep structure are mainly due to a reduction of circadian force. At a neural circuitry level, the reticular activating system that comprises cholinergic, monoaminergic, histaminergic and glutamatergic neurons is responsible for wakefulness, in contrast to the GABAergic neurons that promote sleep [17]. Pathology in the relevant neural substrates may explain insomnia in patients with Parkinson's disease and possibly Alzheimer's disease [19]. Some scholars suggest that monoamines could be the link between REM sleep and depression [20]. However, as with the case of dementia, the exact neural mechanisms between insomnia and mood disorders are yet to be clarified.

In terms of psychosocial aspect, the 3 P models, i.e. predisposing, precipitating, and perpetuating factors, can be used to understand the course of insomnia in elderly people.

#### *3.1.1 Predisposing factors*

As mentioned above, some demographic factors are reported to be related to an increased risk of sleep disturbances. Many of these factors are also predisposing factors for insomnia, including female gender and lower socioeconomic status, and physical and mental health illness [21]. Divorced couples and widowers also have a high prevalence of insomnia [21]. This agrees with the findings mentioned above that loneliness is associated with sleep disturbance [3]. Family history of insomnia, poor sleep hygiene, stress, poor sleep environment, low physical activity level and use of substances are other predisposing factors that clinicians should consider [21–23]. Loss of a spouse and low physical activities are also relevant concerns for elderly people.

#### *3.1.2 Precipitating factors*

New onset or deterioration of medical and mental illnesses can precipitate insomnia in the elderly. Symptoms and worrisome brought by medical diseases can affect sleep quality. Hospitalisation, and certain drug use, such as decongestants and steroids, also precipitate insomnia [23, 24]. Psychological stressors and stressful life events that precipitate insomnia include financial problems, changes in living environment, e.g. moving to nursing homes, and the death of loved ones [24, 25].

#### *3.1.3 Perpetuating factors*

Perpetuating factors are behavioural and cognitive changes that occur after the onset of diseases and prolong an acute insomnia episode into chronic problems [23]. Patients with insomnia may take frequent naps that compensate for short or poor night's sleep. Besides, they may stay awake for a prolonged time in bed due to difficulties falling asleep [23]. These maladaptive behaviour changes can prolong and worsen the problem of insomnia. From the cognitive aspect, patients may be worried or even anxious about not being able to fall asleep, which further worsens insomnia [23]. A vicious circle is formed, and patients may eventually rely heavily on medications to treat insomnia.

### 3.2 Sleep, depression and anxiety

Sleep disturbances, mainly insomnia, are common symptoms of depressive disorders and general anxiety disorder. A recent longitudinal study on middle-aged and older people suggested a bidirectional relationship between short sleep duration and depression [25]. Several other studies also indicated that perceived poor sleep quality correlates with depressive and anxiety symptoms among elderly people [26–28]. Therefore, depression and anxiety are important differential diagnoses for elderly patients who present with sleep disturbance.

#### *3.2.1 Late-life depression*

The presentation of depression in elderly people may be different from that among younger adults. Elderly people may be less likely to complain of low mood than younger adults. In contrast, they may show more irritability, anxiety and somatic symptoms [29]. Also, non-demented elderly patients with depression may present like cognitive impairments [30]. Indeed, a close relationship between depression and cognitive functions in elderly people has been reported. Depression is found to be associated with the occurrence and progression of neurocognitive disorder [31, 32]. Physical health-related risk factors of depression among older adults include chronic diseases, especially vascular-related diseases, disability and self-perceived health [33]. Several mechanisms have been proposed to explain the biological basis of late-life depression. The vascular depression hypothesis suggests that cerebrovascular diseases or cerebrovascular risk factors can lead to depression [34]. The hypothesis is supported by imaging studies and the fact that depression is more common in post-stroke patients [29, 34]. The inflammation hypothesis suggests that the persistent activation of microglia and inflammatory response within the brain lead to an imbalance in the cytokines system and subsequently lead to neuronal death and reduced neuroplasticity [34]. Psychological risk factors of depression among elderly people include maladaptive coping strategies and negative self-image [33].

#### *3.2.2 Generalised anxiety disorder*

A recent study done in a multicentre setting suggested that the prevalence of generalised anxiety disorders was about 3.1% in the elderly [35]. Although not all studies suggested a strong co-occurrence between generalised anxiety disorder and depression in the elderly population, there is a high overlap in the symptoms between the two disorders and co-occurrence in the clinical population [35, 36]. Elderly patients with GAD may also present with frequent somatic complaints with unexplained symptoms [36]. The biological and psychological risk factors of anxiety and depression show significant similarities [33]. It has also been suggested that elderly patients with GAD may progress to depression [36, 37]. Therefore, the clinician should screen for depression in patients the present with symptoms of generalised anxiety disorder, including sleep disturbances. Deteriorated physical health and life events can lead to worrying in elderly people. Clinicians need to identify excess, uncontrollable and unrealistic worrying of elderly people that may suggest anxiety disorders [36].

## 4. Neurocognitive disorders

The decline in cognitive functions is common among the elderly population. Mild cognitive impairment (MCI) refers to a syndrome where one's experiences cognitive decline more significant than expected with regard to one's age and education while activities of daily living are not notably interfered with [38]. Dementia, in contrast, refers to a great extent of cognitive decline severe enough to affect daily living [38].

Sleep problems are common in people with MCI and dementia, particularly in patients with Alzheimer's disease (AD) and Lewy body dementias (LBD) [39]. The elderly with different types of dementia may present with different kinds of sleep disturbance. Sleep disturbance is a predictor of more severe cognitive and neuropsychiatric symptoms and poorer quality of life [39]. However, it does not mean that the longer the sleep duration, the better for the demented patients. Indeed, results from a meta-analysis suggest that too short (i.e. less than 5 hours) and too long sleep duration (i.e. longer than 9 hours) also correlated with the poor cognitive performance of various domains, including executive function, as well as verbal and working memory [40].

### 4.1 Alzheimer's disease

Alzheimer's disease is the most common and well-known cause of dementia worldwide [41]. Pathogenesis of the diseases involved amyloid plaque and neurofibrillary tangle formation that is associated with neuronal loss and cognitive decline in affected patients [42]. Common psychiatric symptoms are apathy, followed by depression, aggression, anxiety and sleep disorder [43]. Of note, about 40% of AD patients experience sleep disorders [43].

Sleep problems of people with AD can present in different ways. One of the common presentations is significant sleep fragmentation, i.e. more frequent and longer period of intra-sleep wakefulness [44]. Although awakening is not the most common sleep disturbance among AD patients, it brings the most disturbance to caregivers [45]. Factors associated with night-time awakening include male gender, more severe memory and functional deficit [45]. Other sleep problems include daytime sleepiness and early morning weakness [44, 45]. Some patients experience a shift in sleep–wake rhythm; in extreme cases, the patients may exhibit day/night sleep pattern reversal [46]. However, in end-stage AD, patients may appear to sleep throughout the day with brief periods of awakening [46].

Sundowning, referring to an increase in behaviour disturbances in demented patients late in the day, is common among patients with AD [46]. Sundowning can begin in the later afternoon or early evening. Sundowning behaviour includes agitation, reduction in attention, disorganised speech, motor disturbance like wandering, hallucinations and emotional disturbances, e.g. anxiety and anger [46]. Sundowning itself reflects a disturbed diurnal rhythm of the affected patients, and improving the nocturnal sleep problem of the patients may alleviate the symptoms of sundowning [46].

Studies have also suggested that altered sleep duration, sleep fragmentation and insomnia are associated with risk of MCI and AD [39]. Although it is not sure whether sleep disturbance is an early marker of cognitive impairment, or causes cognitive impairment, good sleep seems to be a protective factor against AD [39].

### 4.2 Lewy body dementias

Lewy body dementias refers to dementia with Lewy bodies (DLB) and Parkinson's disease dementia (PD-D) [47]. Hypersomnia is common in patients with Lewis body dementias due to nocturnal sleep fragmentation, sleep apnea, periodic limb movement and change in sleep–wake physiology [47]. For PD-D, other behavioural features associated with PD-D include apathy, loss of motivation, change in personality and psychosis [48]. Visual hallucinations are more common than other sensory modalities of hallucination and are usually complex, e.g. seeing people, objects and animals [48]. Delusions are usually paranoid in nature or phantom border [48].

The clinical features of DLB and PDD are similar. Similar to PD-D, patients with DLB may also experience detailed and well-formed visual hallucinations of people, animals or objects [49]. DLB patients may present with daytime drowsiness and disorganised speech [49]. Fluctuations in cognition, attention and arousal are typical characteristics of DLB [49]. A core features of DLB are REM sleep behaviour disorder (RBD) which may precede cognitive decline [49]. RBD can lead to significant injuries that require hospitalisation, yet its prevalence may have been underestimated [50].

### 4.3 Sleep-disordered breathing and cognitive impairment

Both obstructive and central sleep apnea prevalence increase with age [51, 52]. The prevalence of sleep-disordered breathing (SDB) is higher in men than women, yet the difference disappears in the elderly age group [52, 53]. Cognitive impairments are also common in patients with sleep-disordered breathing. Studies suggested that obstructive sleep apnea is associated with neurodegeneration and pathological process closely related to Alzheimer's disease [53]. A study done in a multicentre setting in Italy also showed that around 60% of patients with different degrees and types of neurocognitive impairments had SPD [54]. In fact, elderly people with obstructive sleep apnea are associated with a range of medical conditions in addition to cognitive decline. These medical conditions include cardiovascular diseases, stroke, chronic pulmonary diseases and depression [55]. While the metabolic mechanisms behind it are not well defined, OSA leading to intermittent hypoxemia, followed by sympathetic activation, sleep fragmentation and sleep deprivation, are believed to be part of the reasons. Diagnosis of OSA in elderly patients is easily missed, partly due to the non-specific symptoms. Some of these presentations are common in elderly people without OSA, including nocturia, gait disturbance, and post-operative delirium. Other symptoms may mimic other neurological and psychiatric conditions, including limb movement during sleep, fragmented sleep, mood disturbance and daytime attention.

While daytime sleepiness is one of the key presentations of OSA, studies have shown that daytime sleepiness is less common among elderly patients compared with younger patients [56]. Although continuous positive airway pressure (CPAP) has been proven to be effective in improving symptoms of OSA, its acceptance among elderly patients is reported to be low. Studies in Asia showed that CPAP is not accepted by a majority of elderly patients [57, 58].

## 5. Medical diseases and sleep disturbance

Multimorbidity is a characteristic of patients in the older age group. Medical diseases can lead to sleep disturbance in several ways. Symptoms of medical diseases disturb sleep (**Table 1**). Besides, medical diseases can precipitate mood disorders that further worsen sleep problems. Sleep problems, in turn, can worsen disease outcomes. Examples include stroke [62], diabetes mellites [64] and cardiovascular diseases [65]. The relationships among medical disease, mental illness and insomnia can be complex. One example is chronic pain in elderly people. Chronic pain is common in elderly people. Chronic pain can directly lead to sleep and psychological distress. Studies suggested that chronic pain is strongly associated with depressive and insomniac symptoms among the elderly [66, 67]. On the other hand, patients with depressive symptoms with or without insomnia are more likely to experience distress from pain [67]. A more recent study that looked into the temporal relationship between insomnia and chronic pain suggested that insomnia could be a risk factor for chronic musculoskeletal pain, with depressive symptoms bearing a partial mediating effect [68].

| System | Disease | Symptoms/conditions contributing to sleep problems |
|---|---|---|
| Cardiovascular | Heart failure | • Nocturnal<br>• Orthopnea<br>• Paroxysmal Nocturnal Dyspnea |
| Respiratory | Asthma [59] | • Nocturnal exacerbation [55] |
| | Chronic obstructive pulmonary disease [60] | • Increase arousal [60]<br>• Nocturnal cough [60]<br>• Obstructive sleep apnea [60] |
| Neurological | Parkinson's disease [61] | • Vivid dreams related to drug treatment [61]<br>• Motor symptoms, including restless leg syndrome and periodic leg movement<br>• nocturia [61]<br>• akinesia leading to difficulties in turning in bed [61] |
| | Stroke [62] | • Sleep-disordered breathing [62]<br>• Sleep–wake cycle disturbances [62] |
| Gastroenterological | Gastroesophageal reflux disease [63] | • Nocturnal [63] gastroesophageal reflux<br>• gastrophagitis [63] |
| Endocrine | Diabetes mellites [64] | • Nocturia<br>• Congestive heart failure [64]<br>• Neuropathy and pain [64]<br>• Obstructive sleep apnea [64]<br>• Restless leg syndrome [64]<br>• Nocturnal hypoglycaemia [64] |

| System | Disease | Symptoms/conditions contributing to sleep problems |
|---|---|---|
| Urogenital | Chronic kidney failure | • Nocturia<br>• Uremia |
| Musculoskeletal | Chronic musculoskeletal pain | — |

**Table 1.**
*Common medical diseases and related symptoms or conditions in elderly people that disturb sleep.*

Elderly patients may not volunteer sleep problems when seeing doctors for medical diseases. For the sake of holistic care and a better outcome for medical diseases, sleep problems should be considered to ask during consultation for relevant elderly patients, especially in primary care settings.

## 6. Delirium

Delirium refers to an acute deterioration of attention, cognition and consciousness. Delirium is common in elderly people in admission, especially in the ICU setting [69]. While old age is a predisposing factor for delirium, older adults can bear multiple predisposing factors that make them vulnerable to delirium. These predisposing factors include underlying cognitive impairment, sensory deficits, comorbidities and low functional state [70]. Common precipitating factors for delirium include medication, particularly polypharmacy and use of psychoactive drugs, infection, bladder catheter, electrolytes and metabolite disturbance, trauma and surgery [70]. Sleep and delirium are highly related. One of the key supporting features of delirium sleep–wake cycle disturbance, while sleep deprivation can predispose to delirium [69, 70]. Poor sleep environment and circadian misalignment in hospitals therefore can contribute to delirium in elderly people in admission [69]. Drug choice for delirious patients is important. Opioids, sedating and hypnotic drugs, including benzodiazepine and anticholinergic, can precipitate delirium [69, 70]. Although antipsychotic and sedative drugs may reduce agitation and behavioural symptoms of patients, these medications may turn patients with hyperactive delirium into hypoactive delirium [70]. Hypoactive delirium tends to be under-recognised by clinicians and has poor survival outcomes [70, 71]. Therefore, non-pharmacological treatment and reduction of the insulting drugs should always be considered first and maximised in delirious patients [69, 70].

## 7. Clinical approach

### 7.1 Diagnosis and screening

The rest of the chapter focus on the clinical approach and management of older adults with sleep disturbance. The general clinical approach for sleep disorders in elderly is illustrated in **Figure 1**. Sleep complaints can be related to 1) sleep pattern, 2) quantity, 3) sleep quality and 4) underlying causes for sleep disturbance.

1. Sleep pattern Sleep: Disturbance can occur at different time points throughout sleep. Starting from the onset of sleep, elderly people may complain of advanced

*DOI: http://dx.doi.org/10.5772/intechopen.111656*

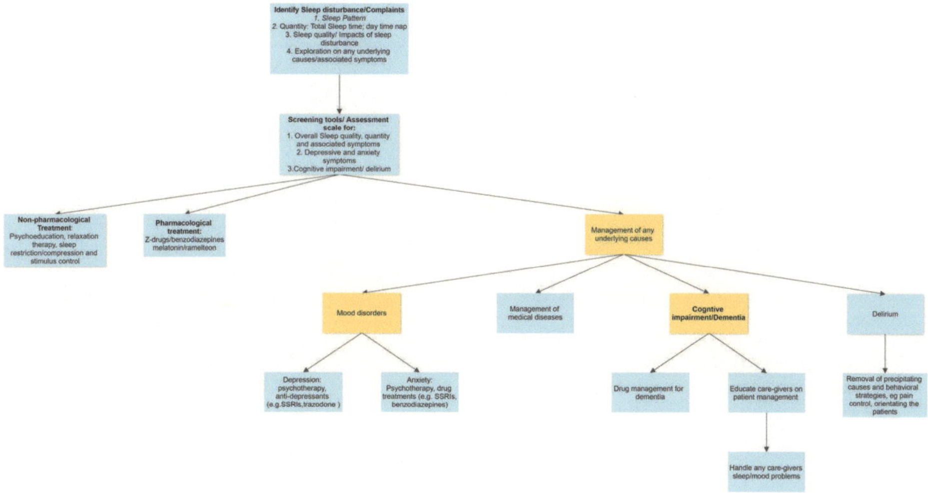


**Figure 1.**
*General approach for elderly people with sleep disturbance.*

or delayed sleep phase syndrome. Some elderly people may even show a day-night reversal sleep pattern or stay awake for most of the night. Elderly patients may experience sleep latency, i.e. difficulty in falling asleep. In the middle of sleep, patients may experience difficulties in maintaining sleep and easy awakening, i.e. sleep fragmentation. Towards the end of sleep, early morning awakening can signify neurocognitive disorders or mood disorders.

2. Quantity: Older adults may have short night sleep or total sleep time. On the contrary, some older adults may complain of hypersomnolence or increased time on napping during the daytime.

3. Quality of sleep and effects on daily living: Some older adults may complain of non-refreshing sleep, resulting in daytime sleepiness or prolonged day sleeping. Sleep problems can relate to reduced concentration, mood disturbance, poor memory, falls and a decrease in daily functions [24].

4. Underlying causes of sleep disturbance. For patients suffering from insomnia, identify the 3-P (see above.) Signs and symptoms of mood disorders and medical diseases that can lead to sleep disturbance, if any, should also be explored. Patients' spouses or caregivers can also be asked for any snoring, witness apnea, limb movement or parasomnia of the patients.

Several screening tools can be considered for symptom evaluations (**Table 2**).

## 7.2 Non-pharmacological management

### 7.2.1 Non-pharmacological Management for Insomnia

A wide range of management options for insomnia is listed in **Table 3**. Several non-pharmacological managements can be considered in elderly patients with insomnia. Cognitive behavioural therapy for insomnia (CBT-I) is recommended as a first-line treatment for chronic insomnia [82]. CBT-I should also be always considered for

| Aim/Objective | Screening tools | Remarks |
|---|---|---|
| Screening for sleep disturbance factors | Global sleep assessment questionnaire | Comprehensive and relatively brief [72] |
| Assessing daytime sleepiness | Epworth Sleepiness Scale | Correlated well with symptoms of OSA [73] |
| Assessing sleep quality and quantity | Pittsburgh sleep quality index | Correlated with psychological symptoms in middle age and older adults [74] |
| Screening symptoms of anxiety and depression | Hospital Anxiety and Depression Scale | Possible ceiling effect, but adequate for the general older population [75] |
| Assessing the severity of depressive syndromes | Hamilton rating scale for depression | Need trained interviewer; for patients with depression disorders [76] |
| Screening elderly people with depression | Geriatric Depression Scale | Several forms with different lengths available; have high sensitivity and specificity [77] |
| Screening anxiety symptoms | Geriatric Anxiety Inventory | Validated for elderly people, available in several languages [78] |
| Identifying cognitive impairments | Montreal Cognitive Assessment (MoCA) | Measure various cognitive domains |
| | Mini-Mental State Examination | Ceiling effect copy right issue Shorter |
| Identifying delirium | Confusion Assessment Method | Widely used in clinical settings with good sensitivity [70] |
| Screening for REM sleep behaviour disorder | REM sleep behaviour disorder screening questionnaire | High sensitivity but relatively low specificity [79] |

**Table 2.**
*Screening tools for elderly people with sleep problems.*

elderly patients, yet, there are more challenges during implementation and flexibility is required [81]. CBT -I consist of psychoeducation, relaxation therapy, cognitive therapy and behavioural strategies, which include sleep restriction and stimulus control [82]. For sleep education, elderly patients should be advised to construct a daily sleep routine and avoid going to bed too early [81]. As mentioned before, the sleep advancement phase is common in elderly people, partly due to psychosocial reasons. Elderly people be encouraged to set a sleep schedule to prevent going to bed too early. A comfortable and suitable sleep environment is essential. For hospitalised or institutionalised elderly people, sleep disruptions from the sleep environment should be minimised. Night-time lighting, bed restraints, TV noise or interference from other patients are common causes that disturb wards or nursing home sleep environments [81, 85]. For patients staying in nursing homes, caregivers can decorate the sleep environments with objects that elderly people are familiar with [85]. For example, elderly people can bring their own pillows, blankets or other personal belongings with them to nursing homes [85]. Lifestyle changes imported for elderly people include ensuring regular daytime physical activities and avoiding prolonged napping [81, 85]. For stimulus controls, elderly patients should not stay in bed or bedroom in case of difficulties in falling asleep. However, due to pain or immobility, implementing stimulus control can be difficult [81]. Sitting up patients, listening to music, reading and other non-stimulating activities can be carried out instead [81]. Similarly, sleep restriction is effective but difficult to be carried out in institutionalised elderly people or those who are ill [81].

| Treatment modalities | Indications | Content/application | Advantage and disadvantage |
|---|---|---|---|
| CBT | Insomnia and related mood disorders | • Sleep hygiene<br>• Maintain activity level<br>• Stimulus control<br>• Sleep restriction<br>• Relaxation therapy<br>• Mindfulness<br>• Cognitive therapy, e.g. avoid secondary worrisome due to insomnia | • No side effects<br>• Help spare sleep medication [80]<br>• Effectiveness may decrease with age [80]<br>• require longer time to take effects<br>• May be less suitable for patients with cognitive impairments<br>• Difficult to implement in bed-bound or institutionalised elderly patients. |
| Light therapy | Insomnia with or without depression; demented patients with sleep–wake disturbance | • Both artificial light or going outdoor can be considered [81]<br>• Patients should be reminded no to look directly into the light source, nor wear sun-glasses during therapy [81]<br>• Light box can be placed in area where elderly people conduct daytime indoor activities [81] | • Little side-effects, if any<br>• Effectiveness not supported by strong evidence [82]<br>• Availability of light sources varies in different institutions<br>• Can be considered as an adjunct therapy [82] |
| Hypnotics Acting on GABA receptors | Insomnia | • Z-drugs, e.g. zopiclone, zaleplon, zolpidem<br>• Benzodiazepines | • Fast and effective<br>• Bring risks of falls and delirium in elderly people<br>• Beware of misuse<br>• Avoid long-term used |
| Anti-depressants | Depression, anxiety disorders and related sleep problems | • SSRI and SNRI can be used for depression and anxiety disorder<br>• Mirtazapine, trazodone and doxepin carry hypnotic effects | • Trazodone may bring serious effects in elderly people, including of orthostatic hypotension, cardiac arrhythmias, priapism and psycho-motor and cognitive impairment [23, 24, 83]<br>• Miratzapine has a good safety profile [84]<br>• Doxepin relatively has few adverse effects on cognitive functions but may have prolong effects on patients with renal impairment |

*CBT = cognitive behavioural therapy; GABA = γ-Aminobutyric acid; SSRI = selective serotonin reuptake inhibitors; SNRI = serotonin and norepinephrine reuptake inhibitors.*

**Table 3.**
*Main treatment choices for elderly people with sleep disturbance.*

Sleep restriction can aim to reduce the total time spent in bed by 20–30 minutes every week to increase sleep efficiency [81]. Cognitive behaviour therapy can also be used to treat underlying mood disorders related to sleep problems. Cognitive sleep therapy can improve symptoms of anxiety disorders [86, 87], although the reported effectiveness varies and is not superior to medication. CBT may also show a decreased effectiveness in elderly patients with anxiety and cognitive impairment [86].

Light therapy has been proposed for elderly people with sleep problems. However, the effectiveness of light therapy on elderly people with sleep disturbance was in doubt. While a systematic review done showed light therapy brings little benefit for elderly people with primary insomnia [80], a more recent meta-analysis supported the efficacy of light therapy in treating geriatric nonseasonal depression [88]. Studies also suggested that bright light therapy can compensate for circadian rhythm alternation in demented patients [89]. However, evidence for light therapy for the treatment of elderly sleep disturbance is not strong and should be considered as an adjunct therapy [82].

#### *7.2.2 Considerations for caregivers of patients with cognitive impairments*

Frontline healthcare professionals should advise caregivers on handling sleep-related problems in elderly people with MCI or dementia. Elderly people with MCI or dementia may wander around at night, even leaving their living place at midnight. The following advice may be helpful for caregivers of these elderly people, for example, their family members [85]: 1. adopting an accepting attitude. Caregivers should avoid direct conflicts with elderly patients. Direct conflicts may agitate the elderly. Instead, caregivers can start the communication with an open-ended question, e.g. "How can I help you with", or "What are you looking for?"; 2. Orienting the elderly patient with environmental cues. Caregivers can show the patients a clock or bring them near the windows to orient them to time; 3. Following the elderly patient and confining the time and place of wandering. Sometimes the patients may exhibit a strong wish to leave their living place for their "home". It may not be easy for caregivers to stop them. In those situations, caregivers will have to follow the elderly patient. The caregivers can try to communicate with the elderly and set an agreed area and duration of wandering.

It is worth mentioning that sleep problems are not only common among elderly patients with dementia, but also among their caregivers. Night-time awakening and short total sleep of patients significantly impair caregivers' sleep [46]. Taking care of demented patients can mount significant mental stress on caregivers. The stress comes from the heavy workload of taking care of the patients and the patient's behaviour disturbances [46, 85]. Therefore, caretakers are prone to mental health problems, including insomnia, comorbid anxiety and depression [85]. Caregivers may present with mood disturbance, somatic complaints, feeling of guilt, suicidal ideation or aggressive behaviours towards the patients [85]. Given that demented patients are often seen together with their caregivers in the clinical settings, frontline healthcare workers should beware of the signs and symptoms of mood disorders of the caregivers [85]. Suitable mental health education and referral should be provided to the caregiver when indicated.

### 7.3 Pharmacological interventions

Although non-pharmacological interventions are preferable because of their minimal, if any, side effects, they do not quickly help patients with sleep problems. Pharmacological interventions have to be considered when sole non-pharmacological interventions do not suffice. Polypharmacy and multiple medical comorbidities are common in older adults and have to be considered when deciding on management plans [24]. Risk-gain balance determines the use of drugs. Fall and cognitive impairments are important considerations for older adults with insomnia treated with drugs. The following provides a brief overview of the general features of common hypnotics on elderly patients. For more details on using of each drug on older people, please view [24].

#### *7.3.1 Z-drugs and benzodiazepine*

A meta-analysis that looked into the effect and adverse drug effects of Z-drugs and benzodiazepines suggested that the effects of sedatives may be diminished in elderly people compared with younger adults [90]. The same meta-analysis also concluded that these sedatives were associated with a higher incidence of falls and likeliness of morning or daytime sleepiness among elderly people [90]. These drugs may impair older adults' balance and cognition and subsequently lead to falls [91]. A higher risk of falls and fractures is related to dose, acting time of agents, concurrent using interacting drugs and time from treatment initiation; that is, 1–2 weeks after treatment initiation is associated with a high risk of falls [91]. Evidence also suggests a higher rate of fracture associated with Zolpidem compared with other benzodiazepines [91].

In elderly patients with severe generalised anxiety disorders and RBD, the use of benzodiazepines is more justifiable [92]. Otherwise, the use of benzodiazepines to treat insomnia should be minimised in elderly people due to the increased sensitivity and decreased metabolism in elderly [92]. Apart from the risk of falls and fractures, benzodiazepine may increase the risk of cognitive decline and delirium [92]. There is also a high risk of misuse of benzodiazepines among elderly patients, who are more vulnerable to the serious effects of benzodiazepine misuse [93]. Benzodiazepine should not be routinely used to treat elderly patients with insomnia [24]. Withdrawal and discontinuation of benzodiazepines should always be considered, given the benefits of doing so on the psychical and psychological health of elderly patients [93].

#### *7.3.2 Melatonin and Ramelteon*

Melatonin may be considered a safer alternative to benzodiazepines in some patients as melatonin is believed not to cause withdrawal and dependence symptoms [94]. Ramelteon is a melatonin receptor agonist, which has been shown to be effective for older adults with chronic insomnia in different studies, particularly for those with difficulties in falling asleep [24, 95]. There is also evidence suggesting ramelteon may help prevent delirium in medically ill elderly people [96].

#### *7.3.3 Other drugs for insomnia*

Some other drugs are used to treat insomnia. Diphenhydramine also provides a sedative effect; however, the possible strong adverse effects in elderly people, including confusion, constipation, dry mouth and cognitive decline in long-term use, suggested that diphenhydramine should not be used for chronic insomnia [24, 92]. Suvorexant is an orexin receptor antagonist that was approved in the USA and Japan for treating insomnia at doses of 10–20 mg [97]. There is evidence suggesting no association between cognitive, psychomotor performance and drug usage at therapeutic dose [98]. Nevertheless, it is still recommended that patients of this drug should take driving precaution and monitoring of apnea-hypopnea index in case of sleep apnea [24].

#### *7.3.4 Drugs for mood disorders, dementia and delirium with sleep problems*

Several antidepressants have been used to treat anxiety disorders and depression in elderly patients. Selective serotonin reuptake inhibitors (SSRIs) and serotonin and norepinephrine reuptake inhibitors (SNRIs) are the mainstay of treatment for late-life anxiety disorders, while benzodiazepines are for patients with severe anxiety [86, 92, 99]. Effective SNRIs for treating anxiety disorders in the elderly include venlafaxine, duloxetine, desvenlafaxine, vortioxetine and mirtazapine [99]. Particularly, mirtazapine carries sedating effect and also can increase patients' appetite [84, 99]. Mirtazapine is thought to be a safe option for elderly patients due to its low cardiotoxicity and no significant changes in vital signs when compared with the placebo group [84]. However, compared with younger adults, older adults on mirtazapine may have a higher chance of experiencing dry mouth, constipation and dizziness [84]. In addition to mirtazapine, trazodone and doxepin are also antidepressants that help insomnia. Use of trazodone in the elderly requires particular cautions due to risks of orthostatic hypotension, cardiac arrhythmias, priapism and psychomotor and cognitive impairment [23, 24, 83]. Doxepin, a tricycle antidepressant, can help elderly people with sleep maintenance [23, 24]. It has few adverse effects on memory and cognitive function [24]; however, reduced clearance of the drug in elderly people with low reduced renal functions may lead to prolonged sedation [24].

Some of the drugs mentioned above are also used in AD patients with insomnia, including low-doze trazodone, mirtazapine and melatonin [39]. Drugs with anticholinergic activities, including antihistamines and tricyclic antidepressants, may exacerbate cholinergic abnormalities and should be avoided in treating elderly patients with AD and insomnia [46, 100]. For patients with LBD, hypersomnia in Lewis body dementia can be treated with modafinil, although some researchers may consider the supporting evidence not strong [47]. Insomnia can be treated with low doses of melatonin [47]. Mirtazapine may exacerbate REM sleep behaviour disorder [47]. lBD patients with autonomic dysfunction may experience orthostatic hypotension, and head elevation during sleep may be needed [47].

Antipsychotics are used in demented elderly patients who are psychotic, severely agitated, aggressive and need drug treatment for sleep [39, 46, 100]. However, the use is controversial due to the possible increase in mortality [39]. For patients with LBD, quetiapine or clozapine is preferred due to their sedative and antipsychotic effects [46]. However, some scholars do not support the use of these antipsychotics in LBD, given little supporting evidence and possible adverse effects on the motor and cognitive of patients. Similarly, use of antipsychotics in patients with hyperactive delirium is also controversial. Some scholars deem the evidence supporting the effectiveness of antipsychotics on delirious elderly people weak [70]. For example, olanzapine may reduce incidence but increase the duration and severity of delirium [70]. Pharmacological treatments in hyperactive delirium for pain relief and sleep enhancement using melatonin are, nevertheless, preferable [70].

## 8. Conclusion

Insomnia is common in elderly people. Identifying underlying psychiatric and medical comorbidities is important for management. Non-pharmacological should always be maximised. Pharmacological treatments are effective, but special cautions are needed to protect elderly people from possible but serious adverse effects, including falls and cognitive decline. Antipsychotics are commonly used in clinical practice for agitated elderly people with dementia and delirium. However, adverse effects may not outweigh the benefits, and limited evidence supports the use of antipsychotics in these patients.

## Conflict of interest

The authors declare no conflict of interest.

## Author details

Pak Wing Cheng* and Yiu Pan Wong
The University of Hong Kong, Hong Kong

*Address all correspondence to: chengpsy@hku.hk

## References

[1] Lu L, Wang S-B, Rao W, Zhang Q, Ungvari GS, Ng CH, et al. The prevalence of sleep disturbances and sleep quality in older Chinese adults: A comprehensive meta-analysis. Behavioral Sleep Medicine. 2018;**17**(6):683-697

[2] Bonanni E, Tognoni G, Maestri M, Salvati N, Fabbrini M, Borghetti D, et al. Sleep disturbances in elderly subjects: An epidemiological survey in an Italian district. Acta Neurologica Scandinavica. 2010;**122**(6):389-397

[3] Smagula SF, Stone KL, Fabio A, Cauley JA. Risk factors for sleep disturbances in older adults: Evidence from prospective studies. Sleep Medicine Reviews. 2016;**25**:21-30

[4] Eguchi K, Hoshide S, Ishikawa S, Shimada K, Kario K. Short sleep duration is an independent predictor of stroke events in elderly hypertensive patients. Journal of the American Society of Hypertension. 2010;**4**(5):255-262

[5] Helbig AK, Döring A, Heier M, Emeny RT, Zimmermann A-K, Autenrieth CS, et al. Association between sleep disturbances and falls among the elderly: Results from the German Cooperative Health Research in the region of Augsburg-age study. Sleep Medicine. 2013;**14**(12):1356-1363

[6] Ohayon MM, Carskadon MA, Guilleminault C, Vitiello MV. Meta-analysis of quantitative sleep parameters from childhood to old age in healthy individuals: Developing normative sleep values across the human lifespan. Sleep. 2004;**27**(7):1255-1273

[7] Schwarz JF, Åkerstedt T, Lindberg E, Gruber G, Fischer H, Theorell-Haglöw J. Age affects sleep microstructure more than sleep macrostructure. Journal of Sleep Research. 2017;**26**(3):277-287

[8] Yaremchuk K. Sleep disorders in the elderly. Clinics in Geriatric Medicine. 2018;**34**(2):205-216

[9] Zepelin H, McDonald CS, Zammit GK. Effects of age on auditory awakening thresholds. Journal of Gerontology. 1984;**39**(3):294-300

[10] Ohayon MM, Vecchierini M-F. Normative sleep data, cognitive function and daily living activities in older adults in the community. Sleep. 2005;**28**(8):981-989

[11] Ancoli-Israel S, Ayalon L, Salzman C. Sleep in the elderly: Normal variations and common sleep disorders. Harvard Review of Psychiatry. 2008;**16**(5):279-286

[12] Foley DJ, Monjan A, Simonsick EM, Wallace RB, Blazer DG. Incidence and remission of insomnia among elderly adults: An epidemiologic study of 6,800 persons over three years. Sleep: Journal of Sleep Research & Sleep Medicine. 1999;**1999**:22

[13] Gulia KK, Kumar VM. Sleep disorders in the elderly: A growing challenge. Psychogeriatrics. 2018;**18**(3):155-165

[14] Swaab DF, Fliers E, Partiman TS. The suprachiasmatic nucleus of the human brain in relation to sex, age and senile dementia. Brain Research. 1985;**342**(1):37-44

[15] American Psychiatric Association. Diagnostic and statistical manual of mental disorders: DSM-5. Arlington, VA: American Psychiatric Association; 2013

[16] Sateia MJ. International classification of sleep disorders-third edition. Chest. 2014;**146**(5):1387-1394

[17] Riemann D, Nissen C, Palagini L, Otte A, Perlis ML, Spiegelhalder K. The neurobiology, investigation, and treatment of chronic insomnia. The Lancet Neurology. 2015;**14**(5):547-558

[18] Cajochen C, Münch M, Knoblauch V, Blatter K, Wirz-Justice A. Age-related changes in the circadian and homeostatic regulation of human sleep. Chronobiology International. 2006;**23**(1-2):461-474

[19] Van Egroo M, Koshmanova E, Vandewalle G, Jacobs HIL. Importance of the locus coeruleus-norepinephrine system in sleep-wake regulation: Implications for aging and alzheimer's disease. Sleep Medicine Reviews. 2022;**62**:101592

[20] Fang H, Tu S, Sheng J, Shao A. Depression in sleep disturbance: A review on a bidirectional relationship, mechanisms and treatment. Journal of Cellular and Molecular Medicine. 2019;**23**(4):2324-2332

[21] Ohayon MM. Epidemiology of insomnia: What we know and what we still need to learn. Sleep Medicine Reviews. 2002;**6**(2):97-111

[22] Morgan K, Clarke D. Risk factors for late-life insomnia in a representative general practice sample. The British Journal of General Practice. 1997;**47**(416):166-169

[23] Patel D, Steinberg J, Patel P. Insomnia in the elderly: A review. Journal of Clinical Sleep Medicine. 2018;**14**(06):1017-1024

[24] Abad VC, Guilleminault C. Insomnia in elderly patients: Recommendations for pharmacological management. Drugs & Aging. 2018;**35**(9):791-817

[25] Sun Y, Shi L, Bao Y, Sun Y, Shi J, Lu L. The bidirectional relationship between sleep duration and depression in community-dwelling middle-aged and elderly individuals: Evidence from a longitudinal study. Sleep Medicine. 2018;**52**:221-229

[26] Chang KJ, Son SJ, Lee Y, Back JH, Lee KS, Lee SJ, et al. Perceived sleep quality is associated with depression in a Korean elderly population. Archives of Gerontology and Geriatrics. 2014;**59**(2):468-473

[27] Paudel ML, Taylor BC, Diem SJ, Stone KL, Ancoli-Israel S, Redline S, et al. Association between depressive symptoms and sleep disturbances in community-dwelling older men. Journal of the American Geriatrics Society. 2008;**56**(7):1228-1235

[28] Yu J, Rawtaer I, Fam J, Jiang M-J, Feng L, Kua EH, et al. Sleep correlates of depression and anxiety in an elderly Asian population. Psychogeriatrics. 2015;**16**(3):191-195

[29] Taylor WD. Depression in the elderly. The New England Journal of Medicine. 2014;**371**(13):1228-1236

[30] Alexopoulos GS. Depression in the elderly. The Lancet. 2005;**365**(9475):1961-1970

[31] Richard E, Reitz C, Honig LH, Schupf N, Tang MX, Manly JJ, et al. Late-life depression, mild cognitive impairment, and dementia. JAMA Neurology. 2013;**70**(3):383-389

[32] Lee ATC, Fung AWT, Richards M, Chan WC, Chiu HFK, Lee RSY, et al. Risk of incident dementia varies with different onset and courses

of depression. Journal of Affective Disorders. 2021;**282**:915-920

[33] Vink D, Aartsen MJ, Schoevers RA. Risk factors for anxiety and depression in the elderly: A review. Journal of Affective Disorders. 2008;**106**(1-2):29-44

[34] Alexopoulos GS. Mechanisms and treatment of late-life depression. Translational Psychiatry. 2019;**9**(1)

[35] Canuto A, Weber K, Baertschi M, Andreas S, Volkert J, Dehoust MC, et al. Anxiety disorders in old age: Psychiatric comorbidities, quality of life, and prevalence according to age, gender, and country. The American Journal of Geriatric Psychiatry. 2018;**26**(2):174-185

[36] Flint AJ. Generalised anxiety disorder in elderly patients. Drugs & Aging. 2005;**22**(2):101-114

[37] Schoevers RA, Deeg DJH, van Tilburg W, Beekman ATF. Depression and generalised anxiety disorder: Co-occurrence and longitudinal patterns in elderly patients. The American Journal of Geriatric Psychiatry. 2005;**13**(1):31-39

[38] Gauthier S, Reisberg B, Zaudig M, Petersen RC, Ritchie K, Broich K, et al. Mild cognitive impairment. The Lancet. 2006;**367**(9518):1262-1270

[39] Wennberg A, Wu M, Rosenberg PB, Spira A. Sleep disturbance, cognitive decline, and dementia: A Review. Seminars in Neurology. 2017;**37**(04):395-406

[40] Lo JC, Groeger JA, Cheng GH, Dijk D-J, Chee MWL. Self-reported sleep duration and cognitive performance in older adults: A systematic review and meta-analysis. Sleep Medicine. 2016;**17**:87-98

[41] Barker WW, Luis CA, Kashuba A, Luis M, Harwood DG, Loewenstein D, et al. Relative frequencies of alzheimer disease, Lewy body, vascular and frontotemporal dementia, and hippocampal sclerosis in the State of Florida Brain Bank. Alzheimer Disease and Associated Disorders. 2002;**16**(4):203-212

[42] DeTure MA, Dickson DW. The neuropathological diagnosis of alzheimer's disease. Molecular Neurodegeneration. 2019;**14**(1):1-18. DOI: 10.1186/s13024-019-0333-5

[43] Zhao Q-F, Tan L, Wang H-F, Jiang T, Tan M-S, Tan L, et al. The prevalence of neuropsychiatric symptoms in alzheimer's disease: Systematic review and meta-analysis. Journal of Affective Disorders. 2016;**190**:264-271

[44] Bombois S, Derambure P, Pasquier F, Monaca C. Sleep disorders in aging and dementia. The Journal of Nutrition, Health & Aging. 2010;**14**(3):212-217

[45] McCurry SM, Logsdon RG, Teri L, Gibbons LE, Kukull WA, Bowen JD, et al. Characteristics of sleep disturbance in community-dwelling alzheimer's disease patients. Journal of Geriatric Psychiatry and Neurology. 1999;**12**(2):53-59

[46] Vitiello MV, Borson S. Sleep disturbances in patients with Alzheimer's disease. CNS Drugs. 2001;**15**(10):777-796

[47] Walker Z, Possin KL, Boeve BF, Aarsland D. Lewy body dementias. The Lancet. 2015;**386**(10004):1683-1697

[48] Emre M, Aarsland D, Brown R, Burn DJ, Duyckaerts C, Mizuno Y, et al. Clinical diagnostic criteria for dementia associated with parkinson's disease. Movement Disorders. 2007;**22**(12):1689-1707

[49] McKeith IG, Boeve BF, Dickson DW, Halliday G, Taylor J-P, Weintraub D,

et al. Diagnosis and management of dementia with Lewy bodies. Neurology. 2017;**89**(1):88-100

[50] Chiu HF, Wing YK, Lam CW, Li SW, Lum CM, Leung T, et al. Sleep-related injury in the elderly—An epidemiological study in Hong Kong. Sleep. 2000;**23**(4):1-5

[51] Bixler EO, Vgontzas AN, Have TT, Tyson K, Kales A. Effects of age on sleep apnea in men. American Journal of Respiratory and Critical Care Medicine. 1998;**157**(1):144-148

[52] Launois SH, Pépin J-L, Lévy P. Sleep apnea in the elderly: A specific entity? Sleep Medicine Reviews. 2007;**11**(2):87-97

[53] Daulatzai MA. Evidence of neurodegeneration in obstructive sleep apnea: Relationship between obstructive sleep apnea and cognitive dysfunction in the elderly. Journal of Neuroscience Research. 2015;**93**(12):1778-1794

[54] Guarnieri B, Adorni F, Musicco M, Appollonio I, Bonanni E, Caffarra P, et al. Prevalence of sleep disturbances in mild cognitive impairment and dementing disorders: A Multicenter Italian clinical cross-sectional study on 431 patients. Dementia and Geriatric Cognitive Disorders. 2012;**33**(1):50-58

[55] Faverio P, Hospenthal A, Restrepo MI, Amuan ME, Pugh MJV, Diaz K. Obstructive sleep apnea is associated with higher healthcare utilization in elderly patients. Annals of Thoracic Medicine. 2014;**9**(2):92

[56] Iannella G, Maniaci A, Magliulo G, Cocuzza S, La Mantia I, Cammaroto G, et al. Current challenges in the diagnosis and treatment of obstructive sleep apnea syndrome in the elderly. Polish Archives of Internal Medicine. 2020;**130**(7-8):649-654. DOI: 10.20452/pamw.15283

[57] Yang M-C, Lin C-Y, Lan C-C, Huang C-Y, Huang Y-C, Lim C-S, et al. Factors affecting CPAP acceptance in elderly patients with obstructive sleep apnea in Taiwan. Respiratory Care. 2013;**58**(9):1504-1513

[58] Ng SSS, Chan T-O, To K-W, Chan K, Ngai J, Ko F, et al. Prevalence of obstructive sleep apnea syndrome and CPAP adherence in the elderly Chinese population. 42 Sleep and Control of Breathing. 2015;**10**(3):1-15. DOI: 10.1183/13993003.congress-2015.pa2342

[59] Luyster FS, Teodorescu M, Bleecker E, Busse W, Calhoun W, Castro M, et al. Sleep quality and asthma control and quality of life in non-severe and severe asthma. Sleep & Breathing. 2011;**16**(4):1129-1137

[60] McNicholas WT, Verbraecken J, Marin JM. Sleep disorders in COPD: The forgotten dimension. European Respiratory Review. 2013;**22**(129):365-375

[61] Menza M, Dobkin RDF, Marin H, Bienfait K. Sleep disturbances in parkinson's disease. Movement Disorders. 2010;**2010**:25

[62] Khot SP, Morgenstern LB. Sleep and stroke. Stroke. 2019;**50**(6):1612-1617

[63] Oh JH. Gastroesophageal reflux disease: Recent advances and its association with sleep. Annals of the New York Academy of Sciences. 2016;**1380**(1):195-203

[64] Surani S. Effect of diabetes mellitus on sleep quality. World Journal of Diabetes. 2015;**6**(6):868

[65] Wolk R, Gami A, Garciatouchard A, Somers V. Sleep and cardiovascular

disease. Current Problems in Cardiology. 2005;**30**(12):625-662

[66] Patel KV, Guralnik JM, Dansie EJ, Turk DC. Prevalence and impact of pain among older adults in the United States: Findings from the 2011 National Health and Aging Trends Study. Pain. 2013;**154**(12):2649-2657

[67] Wilson KG, Eriksson MY, D'Eon JL, Mikail SF, Emery PC. Major depression and insomnia in chronic pain. The Clinical Journal of Pain. 2002;**18**(2):77-83

[68] Generaal E, Vogelzangs N, Penninx BWJH, Dekker J. Insomnia, sleep duration, depressive symptoms, and the onset of chronic multisite musculoskeletal pain. Sleep. 2017;**40**(1):1-10. DOI: 10.1093/sleep/zsw030

[69] Farasat S, Dorsch JJ, Pearce AK, Moore AA, Martin JL, Malhotra A, et al. sleep and delirium in older adults. Current Sleep Medicine Reports. 2020;**6**(3):136-148

[70] Inouye SK, Westendorp RGJ, Saczynski JS. Delirium in elderly people. The Lancet. 2014;**383**(9920):911-922

[71] Yang FM, Marcantonio ER, Inouye SK, Kiely DK, Rudolph JL, Fearing MA, et al. Phenomenological subtypes of delirium in older persons: Patterns, prevalence, and prognosis. Psychosomatics. 2009;**50**(3):248-254

[72] Klingman KJ, Jungquist CR, Perlis ML. Questionnaires that screen for multiple sleep disorders. Sleep Medicine Reviews. 2017;**32**:37-44

[73] Johns MW. Daytime sleepiness, snoring, and obstructive sleep apnea. Chest. 1993;**103**(1):30-36

[74] Buysse DJ, Hall ML, Strollo PJ, Kamarck TW, Owens J, Lee L, et al. Relationships between the Pittsburgh Sleep Quality Index (PSQI), Epworth Sleepiness Scale (ESS), and clinical/polysomnographic measures in a community sample. Journal of Clinical Sleep Medicine. 2008;**04**(06):563-571

[75] Djukanovic I, Carlsson J, Årestedt K. Is the hospital anxiety and depression scale (HADS) a valid measure in a general population 65-80 years old? A psychometric evaluation study. Health and Quality of Life Outcomes. 2017;**15**(1):1-10. DOI: 10.1186/s12955-017-0759-9

[76] Harrison PJ, Cowen P, Burns T, Fazel M. Shorter Oxford Textbook of Psychiatry. Oxford: Oxford University Press; 2018

[77] Krishnamoorthy Y, Rajaa S, Rehman T. Diagnostic accuracy of various forms of geriatric depression scale for screening of depression among older adults: Systematic review and meta-analysis. Archives of Gerontology and Geriatrics. 2020;**87**:104002

[78] Geriatric Anxiety Inventory (GAI). American Psychological Association. American Psychological Association; [cited 2022 Nov 6]. Available from: https://www.apa.org/pi/about/publications/caregivers/practice-settings/assessment/tools/geriatric-anxiety

[79] Stiasny-Kolster K, Mayer G, Schäfer S, Möller JC, Heinzel-Gutenbrunner M, Oertel WH. The rem sleep behavior disorder screening questionnaire-a new diagnostic instrument. Movement Disorders. 2007;**22**(16):2386-2393

[80] Montgomery PA, Dennis J. A systematic review of non-pharmacological therapies for sleep problems in later life. Sleep Medicine Reviews. 2004;**8**(1):47-62

[81] Richter K, Kellner S, Milosheva L, Fronhofen H. Treatment of insomnia in

elderly patients. Journal for ReAttach Therapy and Developmental Diversities. 2020;**2**:129-138

[82] Riemann D, Baglioni C, Bassetti C, Bjorvatn B, Dolenc Groselj L, Ellis JG, et al. European guideline for the diagnosis and treatment of insomnia. Journal of Sleep Research. 2017;**26**(6):675-700

[83] Mendelson WB. A review of the evidence for the efficacy and safety of trazodone in insomnia. The Journal of Clinical Psychiatry. 2005;**66**(04):469-476

[84] Montgomery SA. Safety of mirtazapine: A review. International Clinical Psychopharmacology. 1995;**10**(Suppl. 4):37-45

[85] Chen XL. Daren zhaoguzhe wu shimian pian [Caregiver of Elder People Book Five Insomnia]. Hong Kong: Daren Liliang Youxiangongsi; 2022

[86] Kim Y-K. Anxiety Disorders: Rethinking and Understanding Recent Discoveries. Vol. 1191. Singapore: Springer Nature; 2020

[87] Hendriks GJ, Oude Voshaar RC, Keijsers GP, Hoogduin CA, van Balkom AJ. Cognitive-behavioural therapy for late-life anxiety disorders: A systematic review and meta-analysis. Acta Psychiatrica Scandinavica. 2008;**117**(6):403-411

[88] Chang C-H, Liu C-Y, Chen S-J, Tsai H-C. Efficacy of light therapy on nonseasonal depression among elderly adults: A systematic review and meta-analysis. Neuropsychiatric Disease and Treatment. 2018;**14**:3091-3102

[89] Roccaro I, Smirni D. Fiat Lux: The light became therapy. An overview on the bright light therapy in alzheimer's disease sleep disorders. Journal of Alzheimer's Disease. 2020;**77**(1):113-125

[90] Glass J, Lanctôt KL, Herrmann N, Sproule BA, Busto UE. Sedative hypnotics in older people with insomnia: Meta-analysis of risks and benefits. BMJ. 2005;**331**(7526):1169

[91] Brandt J, Leong C. Benzodiazepines and Z-drugs: An updated review of major adverse outcomes reported on in epidemiologic research. Drugs in R&D. 2017;**17**(4):493-507

[92] American Geriatrics Society 2019 updated. AGS Beers Criteria® for potentially inappropriate medication use in older adults. Journal of the American Geriatrics Society. 2019;**67**(4):674-694

[93] Airagnes G, Pelissolo A, Lavallée M, Flament M, Limosin F. Benzodiazepine misuse in the elderly: Risk factors, consequences, and management. Current Psychiatry Reports. 2016;**18**(10):1-8. DOI: 10.1007/s11920-016-0727-9

[94] Anghel L, Baroiu L, Popazu C, Pătraș D, Fotea S, Nechifor A, et al. Benefits and adverse events of melatonin use in the elderly (review). Experimental and Therapeutic Medicine. 2022;**23**(3):1-8. DOI: 10.1007/s11920-016-0727-9

[95] Neubauer D. A review of Ramelteon in the treatment of sleep disorders. Neuropsychiatric Disease and Treatment. 2008:69-79. DOI: 10.2147/ndt.s483

[96] Chakraborti D, Tampi DJ, Tampi RR. Melatonin and melatonin agonist for delirium in the elderly patients. American Journal of Alzheimer's Disease and Other Dementias. 2014;**30**(2):119-129

[97] Herring WJ, Connor KM, Snyder E, Snavely DB, Zhang Y, Hutzelmann J, et al. Suvorexant in elderly patients with insomnia: Pooled analyses of data from phase III randomised controlled clinical trials. The American Journal of Geriatric Psychiatry. 2017;**25**(7):791-802

[98] Vermeeren A, Vets E, Vuurman EFPM, Van Oers ACM, Jongen S, Laethem T, et al. On-the-road driving performance the morning after bedtime use of suvorexant 15 and 30 mg in healthy elderly. Psychopharmacology. 2016;**233**(18):3341-3351

[99] Crocco EA, Jaramillo S, Cruz-Ortiz C, Camfield K. Pharmacological management of anxiety disorders in the elderly. Current Treatment Options in Psychiatry. 2017;**4**(1):33-46

[100] Cipriani G, Lucetti C, Danti S, Nuti A. Sleep disturbances and dementia. Psychogeriatrics. 2014;**15**(1):65-74

Section 3

# Innovations in Sleep Technology – Asleep or Awake

Chapter 6

# Reduction of Stress and Jet Lag, Improvement of Well-Being, Sleep Quality and Body-Mind Regeneration by Vinci Power Nap® Neuroarchitecture System: Innovative Solution for Leaders, Employees, Travelers

*Magdalena Filcek and Mayank Vats*

## Abstract

The Vinci Power Nap® system is a cutting-edge tool for reducing stress and jet lag effects associated with air travel, allowing for quick body–mind regeneration and improving well-being and the quality of night's sleep. Power naps in a specially designed environment based on interdisciplinary science, can restore homeostasis and work–life balance, release stress and tensions, strengthens focus and efficiency, and recover energy for life to many overtired leaders, employees, and people with sleep disorders. Helpful in the therapy for hypersensitive people, after trauma, in depression, with oncological experiences, and many other diseases. The research made in UN projects at COP24 on leaders, travelers, and UNICEF Ukraine's refugees show extraordinary relaxing properties, harmonizing sleep patterns and internal vital parameters (breath, heartbeat, and brain waves) thanks to zero gravity position, pulsating touch, frequency swinging, calming all senses and neuroarchitectural external conditions. Sleep is the basis of our psychophysical and immune regeneration and preventing errors resulting from stress and fatigue. The Vinci Power Nap® system is crucial for hotels and airports due to its ability to reduce discomfort associated with jet lag, providing great help to travelers such as business leaders, pilots, doctors, drivers, athletes, workers, soldiers, astronauts, tourists, etc.

**Keywords:** sleep, regeneration, energy, efficiency, stress, jet lag, circadian rhythms, wellbeing, astronauts, pilots, tourists, hotels, depression, trauma, PTSD, airports, aviation, neuroarchitecture, Vinci Power Nap®, histamine, antihistamine, enzyme DAO

## 1. Introduction

A high quality night's sleep is the basic element enabling the harmonious and efficient functioning of the body and mind during the day, which strengthens overall health, well-being, and productivity and plays a huge role in memory consolidation and cell rejuvenation. Sleep deprivation and stress leads to altered immune function [1] and many diseases, such as increase risk of diabetes, atherosclerosis, and Alzheimer's, among others, very often leading to chronic diseases, frustration, depression, and even suicide; according to prof. A. Perski from Stockholm Stress Clinic, it also may be the cause of cancer. New research shows that a lack of adequate sleep can lead to irreversible DNA damage and cause cancer [2]. The rats prevented from falling asleep, after 3 weeks, died due to systemic inflammatory response syndrome of sepsis [3].

Over 60% of people (children and adults) around the world are currently reporting sleep problems [4, 5]; shift workers, "coronosomnians," and passengers flying long distances, suffering from jet lag, are increasing those numbers [6, 7]. Without sleep, human cognitive abilities and reaction time are very limited. The efficiency of mind decreases significantly; it is difficult to concentrate, and mental work is not possible. The immune system of the body decreases rapidly, and the pain sensations can become more severe. It is also impossible to make rational decisions. A very large number of people do not even realize how lack of sleep reduces the quality and safety of life; the high-risk group includes leaders, businessmen, doctors, drivers, pilots, astronauts, soldiers, travelers, and so on. A 2001 study in the British Medical Journal showed that stressful work, tiredness, and not enough of sleep could double the errors in a doctor's practice [8]. Conclusions from the Biological Rhythms Research Laboratory is that sleep deprivation as well as jet lag symptoms can ruin vacations and impact athletes, musicians, surgeons, and businessmen who are unable to reach their peak [9]. The WHO recognized insomnia and sleep disorders as a disease of civilization that should be treated [10].

Neuroscience and neuroarchitecture advances provide the ability to measure metrics and allow to understand how environmental pollution factors like colors, shapes, smell, light, sounds or silence, changes in electromagnetic field's frequencies, and temperature can affect human perception, emotions, and physiology and even block the way for the best quality of sleep. The same knowledge can be used to change those parameters for the better, to create neuroarchitectural projects, which could help improve sleep and prevent insomnia [11]. The author conducted survey research on support of stress, trauma, sleep, and jet lag reduction through VPN sessions on 465 UN delegates traveling to Poland for COP24 from 58 countries who participated in VPN sessions during the 14 days of the conference; 127 refugee women and children from Ukraine, who participated in UNICEF project to soothe war trauma; 12 pilots; 41 employees of 3M company; 14 people with depression; and 14 soldiers with PTSD experiencing sleep disorders, through polysomnography and observations on analog astronauts and the author's own experience in reducing symptoms of jet lag after traveling from Poland to Tokyo. The results shows that synchronization and restoring harmony and energy for life after a long journey through several time zones can be possible thanks to the latest neuroarchitecture technology of the Vinci Power Nap® system. The interdisciplinary connections of various sciences in the VPN system interacting with each other during the sessions, and the author's deep researches, allow to understand its mechanisms and supportive aspects for sleep medicine, improving human well-being and psychophysical condition, which is confirmed also by official feedback from participants, psychologists, scientists, and global institutions and ministries.

## 2. The power of sleep and its neuroarchitecture: Asleep or awake

Sleep is a human's superpower—restful deep sleep is time for healing, allowing to regain energy, alertness, focus, creativity, regeneration of physical and mental health, balance homeostasis, and immune system protection, and has antiaging and anticancer properties [12]. "To live well you must sleep well," N.Rothstein The Ambassador of Sleep.

To make good sleep available, many conditions from different science fields that are involved in sleep nature have to be taken into account [13, 14]. This awareness can be helpful to create interdisciplinary designs of neuroarchitecture for better sleep like, for example, the patented Vinci Power Nap® system. Designers, doctors, and solutions engineers should remember that there are connections between external environmental factors (biological, chemical, and physical) and internal body reactions to them. These external factors and internal reactions can increase histamine levels and disrupt regenerative sleep patterns, consequently dictating physical lifestyle and psychological behavioral.

Asleep and awake are strongly connected with the brain, which is an electrochemical organ, and its activity can be measured as brain waves such as gamma, alpha, beta, theta, and delta; each of them has a different rhythm (frequency) and occurs depending also on the day or night activity of the body and mind [15]. The human brain goes through different brain waves in series during the 7–8-hour sleep patterns creating 5 cycles, each cycle lasting 1.5 hours [16, 17] with REM and N-REM stages [18]. The most regenerative rhythm is the deepest frequency called delta waves (0.1–4 Hz) in N-REM; this part of sleep inhibits the nervous system from conducting the impulses from senses, helping to maintain synaptic homeostasis and allowing hemodynamic oscillations of glymphatic fluid clean beta-ameloids (toxic effects of metabolic transformation) from the brain [19, 20]. The changes in delta wave activity and sleep disorders can lead to Parkinson's, Alzheimer's disease, schizophrenia, narcolepsy [21] chronic illnesses, depression, and so on [22].

There are factors that prohibit the brain from entering this regenerative delta waves, like not enough of melatonin hormone [23] (which synthesis from serotonin and can be disrupted by light's smog, blue light, and also lack of serotonin [24]) and the lack of oxytocin hormone, which occurs from not having hugs and pressure on skin. Also, external factors perceived as stressful by human senses, like too high or too low temperature; noise; light; pressure; metals; chemical; toxic ingredients in food, in water, and in air; and electromagnetic fields, can activate the reaction of mast cells to release histamine [25]. In the case of histamine intolerance, it is mainly heavy metals such as mercury, palladium, cadmium, lead and nickel, as well as wood preservatives, mold, pesticides, and car exhaust fumes, which can contribute to the emergence and development of the disease, which highlights the relationship between pollution environment and histamine intolerance.

Histamine as a hormone, as well as a neurotransmitter, strongly participates in the sleep–wake cycle, because an increase in the amount of histamine significantly hinders the process of falling asleep, and thus, blocking the histamine receptors in the brain causes drowsiness; one of the symptoms of histamine intolerance are problems with falling asleep and maintaining deep, restorative sleep [26]. In addition, histamine can open the blood–brain barrier [27]; changes in histamine levels in the brain are closely related to the central nervous system abnormality or impairment in the function and are believed to contribute to neurological disorders [28–30]. Histamine also can be increased by drugs and chemicals as well as alcohol, caffeine, nicotine, cocaine, opioid, and cannabis [31, 32]; its high level and its receptors H1, H2, H3, and H4 [33] cause inflammations (in the most serious cases leading to sepsis [25]), which decrease delta waves [33–35]. In opposition, ketogenic diets can increase the delta wave [36]. Stress and biological processes within the body as a reaction to the external world, long air flights, as well as climate change factors, make endocrine changes, which play a role in the desynchronization of the body rhythms, homeostasis, and sleep patterns, causing jet lag's effects and prevention from good quality sleep, especially in big cities [37–40]. An overwhelming environment, sleep disorders, lack of night regeneration leading to fatigue, anxiety, burnout, chronic diseases, frustration, aggression, tendency to accidents, addictions, depression, and suicide generate not only economic but also social costs. It is so important to create interiors, at home and in public, to calm the senses, where a person can feel safe and fall in regenerative sleep, disconnect for a while from hectic world. To prevent chronic disease now and in the cities of the future, the best solution and benefit will be to prioritize sleep [40–42].

### 2.1 Melatonin, serotonin, and oxytocin: their connections with environment

Scientific studies have shown that the hormone melatonin acts *via* receptors in the modulation and entrainment of biological and circadian rhythms; is engaged in activating lower brain waves and sleep regulation [43]; plays an important role in suppressing inflammation, neuronal and tissue regeneration, and reproduction functions; strengthens immunity and oncostatic systems, and helps to reduce oxidative stress [44].

Melatonin is strongly connected to serotonin as this neurotransmitter is its precursor [45]. The activator for releasing serotonin, dopamine, noradrenaline, and opioids is oxytocin hormone [46], which is why there is a strong connection between melatonin, serotonin, and oxytocin. The synthesis and secretion of melatonin is affected by and also depends on the sunlight exposure to the eyes retina, as the pineal gland [44] converts the light from electromagnetic waves, as signals from the nervous system, to hormonal signals to create chemical communication between the brain and the body as the answer for environmental factors [47–49]. The serotonin–melatonin daily endocrine rhythm is strongly connected with the daily light cycles, and the top pick of melatonin is during the dark, lowering with daylight [50], but also, new studies show that the production of endogenous melatonin can be activated as an answer to the external environmental factors and changes, which are not related to the light/dark cycle [47, 51, 52]. Advances in this field are presenting that in reality, the circadian network is a multiple oscillator system, discovering that different cells/tissues in isolation have the possibility to manage self-sustained oscillations [53, 54], which raises the possibility that the circadian rhythm in various biological processes may be provided by oscillations resulting from local tissue responses to external factors. Following logically, dyssynchrony could occur using both levels, the inter - organ and between environment and organs, until all rhythm processes reset and adjust again to the new light/dark cycle [55, 56], or some other mechanism occurs that will allow all the internal rhythms of the body to be synchronized with the surrounding frequency, giving a sense of harmony [57].

## 3. Vinci Power Nap®: well-being neuroarchitecture with power to synchronize

Vinci Power Nap®, a patented system awarded the Wellbeing Quality Certificate 2019 for the best place in Poland, recommended by NASA JPL, UN, UNICEF, and so

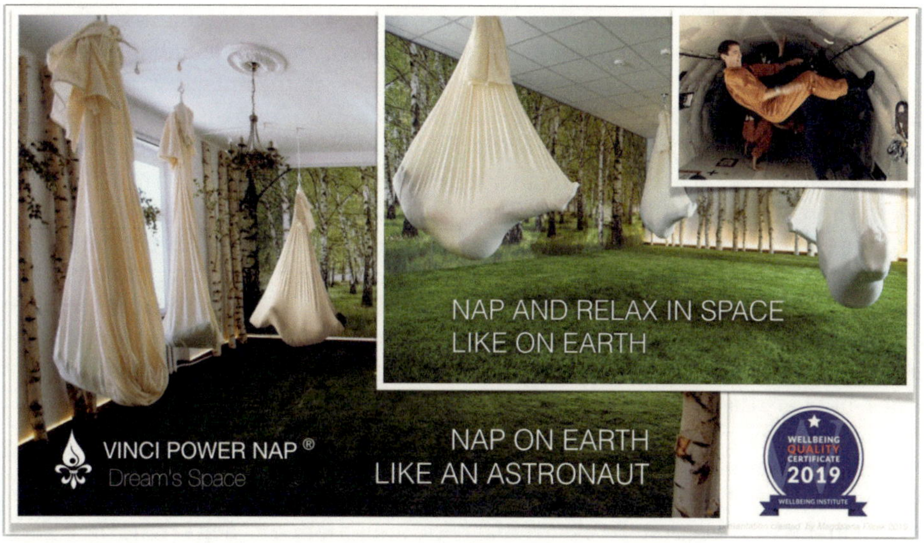


**Figure 1.**
*Patented design interiors of neuroarchitecture of Vinci Power Nap® with human experiencing swinging in zero gravity position, during regenerative session [62].*

forth, is bringing back and giving the best well-being experience for humans. It has been designed by Magdalena Filcek—the pioneer of neuroarchitecture biotechnology mechanisms— as a revolution tool for fast stress reduction and body–mind regeneration [58–61] (**Figure 1**). This experience is possible during 20-min energy naps, while a person laying in zero gravity position in a cocoon, which acts as an oscillation generator, swinging in pendulum movement, in a pollutant-free interior environment, calming all senses at once [39, 63–65]. This pendulum movement is allowing for breath, heartbeat, and brain waves synchronization in special "maternal" frequency 0,618 Hz and 1,618 Hz [40], giving the person feelings of safety and bliss, stress reduction, and rest and sleep with deep relax [39]. The tensions in body muscles can be relaxed thanks to the zero gravity position of the body lying in elastic material of cocoon, feeling suspended, weightless, like in mother's arms.

Swinging in VPN stimulates the vagus nerve, which controls crucial body and mind functions; its activation has the ability to prevent inflammation, rebalance the autonomic nervous system, restore optimal state, and better connect body and mind [66, 67]. The gentle pulsating pressure on skin during cocoon's swinging in calm environment activate also skin receptors (mechanoreceptors and exteroceptors) on biological, chemical, physical and ions levels [68]. This interaction of art and science in VPN designed system and new approach to neuroscience allows the author to find solutions for neurobiological integrations, night sleep improvement, sense of safety/security, work–life balance, well-being, longevity, stress and jet lag reduction, and the connection of internal body clock with surrounding time as a frequency [57].

### 3.1 Vinci Power Nap®: to rest, reset and reconnect human "factory settings"

Resetting and reconnecting the senses with body, mind, and environment in one frequency has been relatively overlooked as until now there was no tool to make it happen. The possibility of "factory settings reset", synchronizing internal human rhythms with external world rhythm, came together with discovering the

Vinci Power Nap® System—as an innovative interdisciplinary mechanism of neuro-architecture that leads to a revolution in sleep medicine and biotechnology.

The electromagnetic field can be found everywhere in the outside world; every ecosystem on the planet from insects to plants, birds, fish, humans, and other living organisms is immersed in the frequency of harmony [57]. Embryonic life, from the first moment in the womb of mother, experiences rhythmic pulsation from the blood flow of mother's vessels that occurs around the placenta, creating the fluctuation of compression and release on the new body in the fetal water—in the rhythm of mother's heartbeat. Following the standards, normal blood pressure is 120–129/80–84 mmHg (dividing 129/80 is ~ 1,618; moreover 80/129 is ~0,618). What is surprising is that the VPN pendulum period is 1.618 s, and at the same time, its frequency shows 0,618 Hz [50]. These two numbers represent the number of Phi, the golden ratio values, but here they are values with Hz forming a harmonic frequency capable of creating 3-dimension fractals [57, 68].

Similar pulsations of contraction and release, compression, and relaxation of the elastic material occur while a person is swinging in the 0,618 Hz gravitational motion in the VPN cocoon. By electromagnetic induction, this delta frequency (0,1 Hz - 4 Hz) from VPN movement occurs in the brain waves, heartbeat and breathing all together at once together with rhythm of environment. Moreover, this pulsation rhythm of pressure on skin triggers the Ruffini and Pacinian receptors to the secretion of hormones like oxytocin and indirectly dopamine, serotonin, melatonin, and so on [69]. The movement of back-forward swinging generates hydrodynamics of fluids in the body, in special rhythm of delta waves, which activate the stimulation of lymphatic [62, 70–71] and glymphatic systems [72], allowing to remove the toxins and neurotoxins [19], cleansing the immune system, increasing activation of enzymes that are able to neutralize histamine [73, 74], and leading to deeper sleep at night [68]. Reducing the level of histamine (also inflammations) and the overabundance of fluid and substances in interstitial is a key for tissue to keep homeostasis [72]. A VPN system can significantly help keep the lymphatic and glymphatic systems running smoothly through the movement of the pulsating rhythm of the pendulum and changing pressure of the cocoon's material. A person, by swinging in this pendulum, can experience weightlessness/microgravity at the highest point, which allows the cells to stretch and absorb water from the tissues, and upon landing to the lowest point, hypergravity occurs, where the cells compress and excess fluid from them that is pumped into the lymphatic system [71]. During this 20-min VPN swinging session, the person falls asleep/naps in a regenerative frequency of delta waves [40]. This process of reset and reconnection is made in the "factory setting" frequency of symmetrical harmony, which rhythm humans can feel physically and mentally pleasant, like in harmoniously combined sounds. The author creates the hypothesis that there is universal rhythm of electromagnetic waves, which feels like gravitation and which is influenced by and interacts with environmental factors and senses with endogenous oscillations, described deeper in article [57]. The ability to synchronize all of the body's internal rhythms with the surrounding frequency can lead to a wonderful feeling of peace, relaxation, rest, bliss, and love, like "coming home," as well as changing the mood and behavior to a more calm and harmonized one, which is exactly what participants say they experience in the VPN session.

The observations from author's research show the importance of the understanding that the biological clock is working with synchrony of the endogenous circadian rhythm together with environmental factors—interacting endocrine systems and human behavior—influencing psychophysical condition. In science, there is a huge progress in understanding chemical and mechanical aspects of cell and tissue, explaining interconnection between the gradients of electromagnetic field (EMF) and cellular reactions, which could be found in research connected with physiology, embryology, and molecular biology—it is showing the correlation between the physical factors and the observed organic, cellular changes [75] together with oscillations of the circadian clock [76] in mammals and plants [77].

## 4. Jet lag and desynchronization of circadian rhythm—Impact for travelers

Jet Lag Disorder (JLD) is mainly connected with long airplane travels, crossing more than 3 time zones [78, 79]; scientists describe it as desynchronization of the internal rhythms of body's internal clock with the rhythm of day and night cycle in the arrived place. Symptoms of jet lag may be different in every person but mainly cause night's sleep problems, tiredness, fatigue and drowsiness during the day, and problems with performance both physical and mental, associated with gastric and somatic issues for few days or even weeks, as described by Stanford University's Center for Sleep Sciences and Medicine [80–82]. According to a study by Eastman published in Sleep Medicine Clinics in 2009, the impact of jet lag on human body is serious and people who fly often can experience long-term health risks and chronic diseases like cardiovascular illness, type II diabetes, and even cancer. This risk is increasing with age following research of the American Academy of Sleep Medicine [9, 82].

The circadian rhythm was found in different kind of organisms as a biological process of endogenous oscillation of hormones, generated by external environment, for example, by temperature, light, and redox in 24-hours cycle. Advances in science show that in living organisms, there are various kinds of clocks, like molecular, chemical, neuronal, and hormonal, where each one is aligned with the others in a bigger or smaller scale [83]; this internal clock regulates body temperature, metabolism, hormone levels, sleep, and behavior [84, 85] and can be disrupted by genetic and/or environmental factors [55, 86].

Hormones' communication is essential for the maintenance of homeostasis and adaptation to environmental changes that stress mast cells into releasing histamine, leading to inflammations [57]. The same stressors are connected with shift work, as the sleep/wake cycle is in this case significantly different from the path of our evolution, where dark and light is in constant and reliable cycle, connected with geophysical patterns. Those disruptions in circadian rhythm have biological consequences and could be linked with higher risk for cancers like colorectal, breast, lymphatic, and prostate, as well as with diabetes, obesity, gastric ulcers, coronary heart disease, atherosclerosis, stroke and heart attack, and so forth [1]. The mechanism for these correlations with exposure to static, flexible, extended, and rotating shift work and frequent international travels by flight crews or travelers across several time zones leads to jet lag symptoms [50]; inflammations and diseases, in author hypothesis, can be connected to mast cells and histamine and its receptors—as pathophysiologic mechanism of sepsis discovered by author and published in [25]. In the complex cycle of sleep and wakefulness, the harmonization of the central histaminergic system plays an important role by promoting and perpetuating the excitability of the cerebral cortex during wakefulness and concentration [1, 73, 87]. The people were defenseless before jet lag as there was no single cure for jet lag [88] and sepsis, until now. The author's research on Vinci Power Nap® allows for understanding the deep connection and interactions between environment, physics, electromagnetic rhythms, and neurobiology/biotechnology of human body, which can give the answer of the mechanism of jet lag and its possible prevention and treatment. This knowledge is a key for any travelers, pilots, astronauts—to let them keep well-being, sleep, and health in better condition and allow to enjoy the trip, work, and vacations.

## 4.1 Stress in the shift work of a pilots, astronauts, flight controllers, and drivers

Specific lifestyle and shift work exposure are connected with circadian and sleep disruptions leading to psychosocial stress. The great responsibility is on the shoulders of the pilots, astronauts, drivers, and flight controllers, as their work is essential to avoid performance errors, but very often, their works' environmental factors, like shift work, huge stress, work overload, noise, changes in temperature (cold or warm), radiation, electromagnetic fields and light intensity, elevated $CO_2$ levels, changes in time zones and gravitational acceleration, vestibular changes, and weightlessness [89–91], are challenging for the body and mind. These environmental stressors lead to the dysregulation of the immune system, multi-organ inflammations, circadian desynchronization, cumulative sleep loss, tiredness, fatigue, and decreased alertness and performance in long-haul flight crews [1]. Moreover, The Center for Disease Control and Prevention classifies airline crew members as "radiation workers" [92, 93] together with ICEMAN project [94]. "The characteristic reaction to electromagnetic radiation consists of tightening in the fascia surrounding the muscles, which in turn causes biochemical failure of the body [75, 95], in particular, disruption of the functioning of cell membranes" [96], changing the probability of ion-channel on/off switching events [97]; this compression, stressful pressure on tissue can active mast cells to release bigger doses of histamine, and its higher level in blood can create clots in the veins (often occurs after flights), causing poor transportation of oxygen to organs, tiredness, headache, sleep disorders, drowsiness, and other symptoms similar to jet lag [98]. Those effects can be very dangerous during airplane flights and space exploration missions [99–103], together with sleep deprivation, which can double error rates [8]; moreover, another study shows that driving tired or sleepy is as dangerous as drunk-driving [104, 105]. Dr. Mark R. Rosekind is Admin. of the National Highway Traffic Safety Administration [106]; his research and reports for NASA show the physiological, psychological effects on flight crews, which are related to stressful flight operations [107]. He has found the operational significance of these effects and presented that effectiveness and operational safety can be lower in the case of the pilot tiredness. He had found that napping is the best operational prevention and the best method to minimize the effects of circadian disruption, sleep loss, and fatigue during the flight operations and has the ability for temporarily reducing stress and physiological sleepiness [108–110]. His studies present that pilots who could take a short power nap increase response time by 54%, in comparison to those who could not take a regenerative sleep during the day; He also notices and provides a very important conclusion: the nap can be shorter but not longer than 26 min [111, 112].

Erin Flynn-Evans, from NASA's Ames Research Center in California's Silicon Valley, is researching how sleep environment disturbances affect the quality of astronauts' sleep during the spaceflight, as astronauts have reported fatigue during missions and deficit of sleep [113]. According to NASA's Human Research Roadmap, there are evidence points to the risk of performance degradation and adverse health effects associated with space exploration missions [114, 115]. The NCAA, in 2016, released a study research of the work environment performed in commercial civilian aviation in Norway, which shows that 72% of pilots and 85% of cabin crew experience physically exhausted after the completion the period of a work [116]. Those high numbers of people with fatigue point to the need for improvement in legislation and real-life practices as "there is an interest in improving both the wellbeing and overall safety of crew, passengers and other relevant stakeholders in the aviation industry" [116]. So far, recommendations have been to report fatigue more often, encouraging people to increase their willingness to report fatigue, try to work less (e.g., 80% instead of 100%), go to bed at decent hours, maintain good sleep hygiene, and allow for napping on the flight deck; a healthy diet and regular physical activity are also very important [116].

The researchers are looking for how to improve performance, determine effectiveness and alertness in flight operations, and plan cockpit rest period and tools.

Great solutions for pilots and astronauts have been found by the author and described broadly in a previous science article titled "Cutting edge solution for effective and safe missions - neuroarchitecture system of Vinci Power Nap® - revolution in fast stress reduction, regenerating body & mind which can help you, pilots, astronauts: before, during and after space travels" [68]. NASA is working to look for the improvements that could increase the astronaut crew's health and prevent illnesses during the spaceflights [117]; following this need, NASA is interested in implementing the VPN system—the innovatively designed environment for fast human regeneration. On May 20, 2019, Manager of NASA JPL/Caltech—Mr. Artur Chmielewski—wrote that he hopes to open the rooms with VPN systems in all NASA centers [118].

### 4.2 Vinci Power Nap® rhythm—The discovery of stress and jet lag relief

The study shows that VPN system can bring remarkable effects regarding relief from stress and jet lag, as it helps in the synchronization of the internal clock with the environment rhythm at the journey destination. Better effects to help for overcoming jet lag symptoms, stress, and tiredness can be achieved by using VPN system as soon as possible after arrival—at the airport or in the hotel. Power nap, in the best calming body and mind environment in zero gravity position, allows not only to sleep deeply and to reduce stress and tensions but also swinging in VPN cocoon with 0,618 Hz frequency during the relaxing session that can, from a biotechnological point of view, help to accelerate enzymatic processes. Research of DSc Lukasz Szymanski, prof. Polytechnic in Lodz, show that the induction of alternating low frequencies of the electromagnetic field can make positive changes in the spin of ferromagnetic atoms, resulting in changes in the properties of some human body substances, such as enzymes, which, in this case, can be helpful in neutralizing the level of histamine, relaxing muscles, faster regeneration of damaged cells, and a positive change in their structure, for instance, increasing the density of bone tissue [119], which is very important prophylaxis for astronauts.

Moreover, during swinging in VPN cocoon, apart from healing activation of vagus nerve [66, 67], the body's active hydrodynamic fluctuations might affect the acceleration of enzymatic catalysis [74] because in the presence of the enzyme, the activation energy for the reaction is less than in its absence; it means that the enzymes can speed up the reaction [74]. For example, swinging in VPN synchronization system [120] for 20 min power nap accelerates enzymes (also as DAO and HMNT) [121], which neutralizes endogenous and exogenous histamine, which can help to prevent and reduce inflammations and its manifestations that are very similar to jet lag symptoms. What showed the pilot research on man 52 years that after 10 VPN sessions, conducted

| ENZYM DAO - BEFORE AND AFTER 10 VINCI POWER NAP® SESSIONS: | | | | |
|---|---|---|---|---|
| Biochemistry before | | | | |
| **Name of study** | **Test result** | **Reference range** | **Reference range** | **sex, age** |
| material: venous blood, serum, date and time. Downloads: 05-06-2023 08:27, date and time admissions: 07/06/2023 11:20 | | | | |
| Diamine Oxidase DAO (serum) | 9,8 U/ml | > 10 | BELOW NORMAL | man 54 years |
| Biochemistry after | | | | |
| Name of study | Test result | Reference range | Reference documents | sex, age |
| material: venous blood, serum, date and time. Downloads: 22-06-2023 08:27, date and time admissions: 26/06/2023 12:24 | | | | |
| Diamine Oxidase DAO (serum) | 15,2 U/ml | > 10 | NORMAL | man 54 years |

**Table 1.**
*Levels of enzyme DAO before and after 10 VPN sessions.*

| VITAMIN D - BEFORE AND AFTER 10 VINCI POWER NAP® SESSIONS: | | | | |
|---|---|---|---|---|
| Immunochemistry before | | | | |
| Name of study | Test result | Reference range | Reference range | sex, age |
| material: venous blood, serum, date and time. Downloads: 05-06-2023 08:27, date and time admissions: 05/06/2023 14:55<br>the tests were performed using the direct chemiluminescence method (CMIA) on the Alinity ci analyzer from Abbott | | | | |
| Vitamin 25(OH)D Total (091) | 28,7 ng/mL | < 20 deficiency<br>20–30 concentration insufficient<br>30–50 optimal concentration<br>50–100 high concentration<br>100–200 potentially toxic concentration<br>> 200 toxic concentration | BELOW NORMAL TOO LOW | man 54 years |
| Immunochemistry after | | | | |
| Name of study | Test result | Reference range | Reference documents | sex, age |
| material: venous blood, serum, date and time. Downloads: 22-06-2023 08:27, date and time admissions: 22/06/2023 13:05<br>the tests were performed using the direct chemiluminescence method (CMIA) on the Alinity ci analyzer from Abbott | | | | |
| Vitamin 25(OH)D Total (091) | 32,4 ng/mL | 30–50 optimal concentration | NORMAL - OPTIMUM | man 54 years |

**Table 2.**
*Levels of vitamin D before and after 10 VPN sessions.*

between June 5, 2023 and June 22, 2023, there was increase of enzyme DAO from 9,8 to 15,2 U/ml (the minimum level of norm is from 10 U/ml); also, the level of vitamin D3 increased from 28,7 to 32,4 ng/mL (the minimum level of norm is from 30 ng/mL) (**Tables 1** and **2**).

The author has hypothesized that neurotechnology of VPN sessions strengthened together with vitamins D3, B6, and C; zinc; enzyme DAO; and antihistamines for H1, H2, H3, and H4 applied before, during, and after the flight or space trip [39] can be a great prevention for pilots, astronauts, and passengers to overcome jet lag, tiredness, and stress, as well as can be helpful in rehabilitation and prevention from organs transplantation rejection [121]. The author has concluded that thanks to VPN system by its identifying the reset mechanism of the internal oscillators and the frequency of hydrodynamic, there is a possibility to balance the endocrine body's interaction on the external environmental factors. This discovery can not only help to bring a better understanding of the circadian biology but also provide insight into more general aspects of controlling biophysics, biochemistry, neurobiology, transplantology, as well flight and space medicine.

### 4.3 Benefits for travelers, pilots, astronauts—Hotel and airport improvement

To not destroy the first days of the vacations or important business negotiation after a long flight trip when few times zones were crossed, to reduce jet lag and improve energy for life, it is recommended to have a 20-minute rest or power nap in Vinci Power Nap® system just after arrival—to reduce symptoms of travel-related body and mind stress [122] and to harmonize the internal rhythm with environmental rhythm at the destination [123].

The best airports and hotels with well-being care for world travelers and their shift-working crew can implement jet lag reduction—reset—energy naps rooms of VPN system as the cutting-edge tool, which is bringing new value in the prevention of human health, as well as performance and energy in space missions.

One part of the VPN system—the cocoon—called the generator of oscillations, is already installed at the AATC (Analog Astronaut Training Center) and is helpful for analog astronauts experiencing sleep deprivation [124]. VPN can be created in spaceships, in future human habitats created on the Moon or on planet Mars. For daytime rest, the author is proposing design of VPN heartbeat frequency pressure cocoon or suit (with changing the pressure on the body in the rhythm of the pendulum VPN movement recorded data from Earth) and for nighttime, a suit with compressed air that exerts gentle pressures on the human body with (0,618 Hz - 1,618 Hz) frequencies, as it is in a mother's womb on Earth [68]—to accelerate the regeneration of cells, release enzymes, and increase bone tissue density [119]. The discoveries of revolutionary properties of VPN system can bring new applications and innovations into sleep medicine, aviation and space medicine, physiology, psychology, and neuroscience.

## 5. The research, subjects, methodology, and results

The author has done interdisciplinary research between March 12, 2018 and January 27, 2023 on hundreds of participants of different groups, showing the real impact of relaxation of VPN sessions on interconnected multilevel human body–mind systems.

The studies were using the measurements for sleep/pulse/brainwaves/heart and HRV tests, laboratory blood, treadmill exercise, and mind performance tests, as well as doctors' and psychologists' deep interviews, surveys, feedback, and observation. Here, only a few from all of the studies are presented, and more are described in another of the author's science articles.

Participants: delegates, leaders, travelers, employees, students, soldiers, pilots, and so on.

### 5.1 Survey on stress and jet lag on Climate Change Conference COP24 2018

The research was done during 14 days of COP24 in Poland, on 465 UN delegates as travelers came from all around the world (different time zones, climate, and culture), suffering also from stress and jet lag. Leaders, 277 women and 179 men, from 58 countries, age range from 15 to 72 years, attended the relaxation session of VPN system. After 20 minutes of VPN sessions, participants filled out the survey, marking their experience and subjective feelings. Based on the results of the data analysis, VPN sessions during COP24 had a significant impact for reducing the symptoms of jet lag in 80% of participants, as decreased fatigue from traveling, relief of stress 98%; bliss and safety 94%; refreshing mind 98%; happy and relaxed 97%, sustainable body and mind 96%; relief from headache and back and neck pain 80%; relief from anxiety 88%; calm/peace, feeling of being loved 96%; and multisensory experience 94% (**Table 3**). The complete survey methodology of research and VPN positive impact on UN delegates is described in [39].

Wellbeing Quality Certificate 2019 — Vinci Power Nap® Dream's Cafe & Dream's Cube *at* COP24 Katowice 2018 United Nations Climate Change Conference

| 465 UN DELEGATES WERE REGENERATED BY VINCI POWER NAP® AT COP24 UNFCCC | |
|---|---|
| ATTENDEE SUMMARY: | |
| **HOW DO YOU FEEL AFTER VINCI POWER NAP® SESSION** | **BETTER** |
| REFRESHING MIND | **98%** |
| SUSTAINABLED / BALANCED BODY & MIND | **96%** |
| RELIEF OF STRESS | **98%** |
| FEELING BLISS & SAFETY | **94%** |
| FEELING HAPPIER & RELAXED | **97%** |
| RELIEVE OF HEADACHE, BACK,NECK PAIN | **80%** |
| RELIEVE OF ANXIETY | **88%** |
| MULTI-SENSORY EXPERIENCE | **94%** |
| FEELING OF CALM/ PEACE AND BE LOVED | **96%** |
| RELIEF OF JET LAG | **80%** |

**Table 3.**
*Results of surveys from 465 UN Delegates on COP24, source: [39].*

### 5.2 UNICEF project: Sleep and stress of women and children with war trauma

The 127 beneficences of UNICEF project for women and children refugees from Ukraine with war stress and trauma attended 300 VPN sessions, a few sessions per person. From 146 filled surveys, the study showed decrease by 86% of the level of stress for 125 people and increase by 87% of the level of feeling safety for 127 people.

The improvement of better night's sleep after the VPN sessions was also reported by UNICEF project participants.

### 5.3 Patterns of sleep and stress for travelers: pilots, soldiers, analog astronauts

There are collected data that show the improvement in fields of sleep, quality increase, and stress reduction for:

**Analog astronauts:** "Analog Astronaut Training Center confirms that the oscillation generator as a part of the Vinci Power Nap® system is used by sleep=deprived analog astronauts as part of their daily routine in the habitat..(...)" Dr. A. Kolodziejczak [124].

**12 international pilots of hot air balloons:** using VPN session in Wroclaw—survey (**Table 4**).

**41 employees of 3M company**: using VPN session in Wroclaw—survey (**Table 5**).

**14 people with depression from clinic**: VPN session in Wroclaw—survey (**Table 5**).

**18 Business Henley School international students**: VPN Wroclaw— survey (**Table 5**).

**14 soldiers with PTSD**: from 10th BkPanc of Polish Army sent by the Ministry of Defense, soldier of special forces GROM, VPN session in Wroclaw—survey (**Table 4**).

**Soldier with PTSD**: deep interdisciplinary physiology, psychology study, and more info about the details of this research are in article [50]. The pilot study on a soldier with PTSD was conducted during 10 days of VPN sessions (everyday session); participant reported increasing quality of refreshing sleep, reducing sense of stress from 10 to 6 level, and unblocking in the senses of smell and taste, and most importantly, he had 2 nights without waking up, which was a big success as flashbacks, insomnia, nightmares, fatigue, recurring thoughts, fears, and so forth were waking him up every night since many years after a war mission, as he reported.

Sleep pilot report of polysonograph conducted on night's sleep of a soldier with PTSD on dates: June 17, 2020 and June 26, 2020; Dr. W. Kucharski from Centrum Serca Lumina Cordis Clinic in Wroclaw, before and after 10 VPN everyday sessions wrote that lever of REM was from 20,13 to 22,45% and deep sleep from 17,56 up to 18,19%; slightly increased RDI (9,3) was recorded with correct AHI (3,2) and ODI (2,8). No sleep apnea was recognized; light sleep dominated as well as correct % of REM sleep (**Figure 2**).

### 5.4 Heartbeat changes after VPN sessions

Heartbeat measurement by pulse oximeter during COP24 on 176 participants and summary chart from the Samsung Health app on a woman experiencing VPN session for the first time. The woman reported serious problems with sleeping before coming to the VPN session; after this session, on the next day (June 26, 2022), she noticed and wrote a comment that she slept 6 hours at night without waking up; it was positively surprising for her because she could not sleep for more than 4 hours every night and it happened for many months before (**Figure 3**).

The results of Holter research before and after 10 VPN sessions showed decreased HR MID from 63 to 60 points and tachycardia from 19 to 8 for the soldier with PTSD

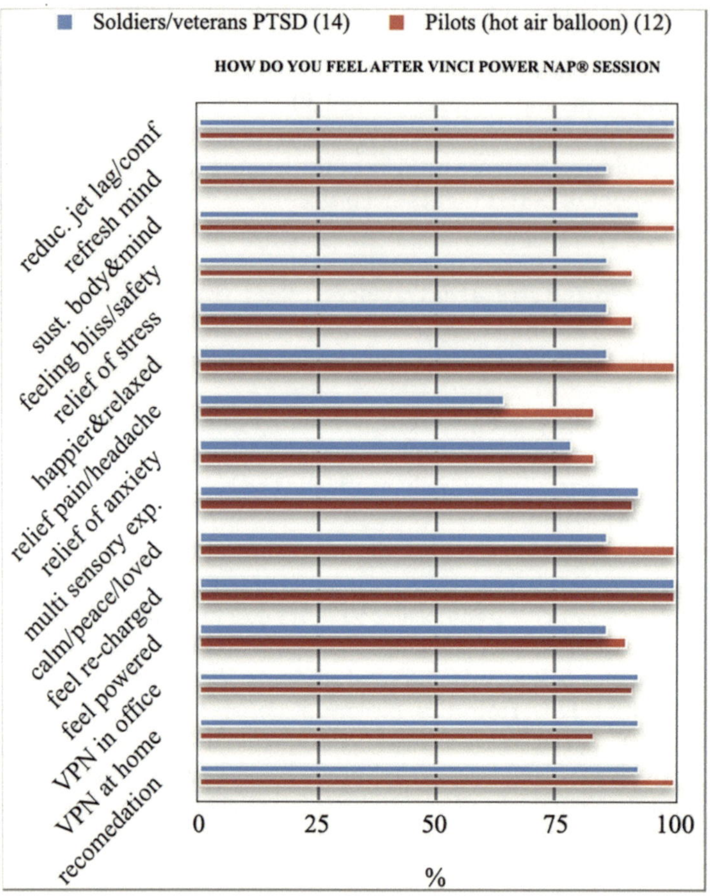


**Table 4.**
*Survey result levels of stress reductions after VPN sessions: Pilots (12) and soldiers with PTSD (14), source [68].*

and HR MID from 88 to 80 points and tachycardia from 1146 to 382 for the woman in trauma, in both increased HRV showing improvement in relaxation. More details of this research are in [40].

### 5.5 Increasing delta waves during the VPN session and rhythm of breathing

During 20 min VPN session for the soldier with PTSD and woman in trauma, the delta and theta waves increased—measured by the neurobiofeedback device, more in [68].

Together with rhythm of VPN movement, the breathing synchronized; rhythm of inhalation and exhalation was with 0,618 Hz frequency in 1,618 s period.

### 5.6 Increasing hormones after VPN sessions

Oxytocin, serotonin, dopamine, prolactin, and testosterone serum increased after VPN sessions—the data and other hormones can be found in study [40] and in [68].

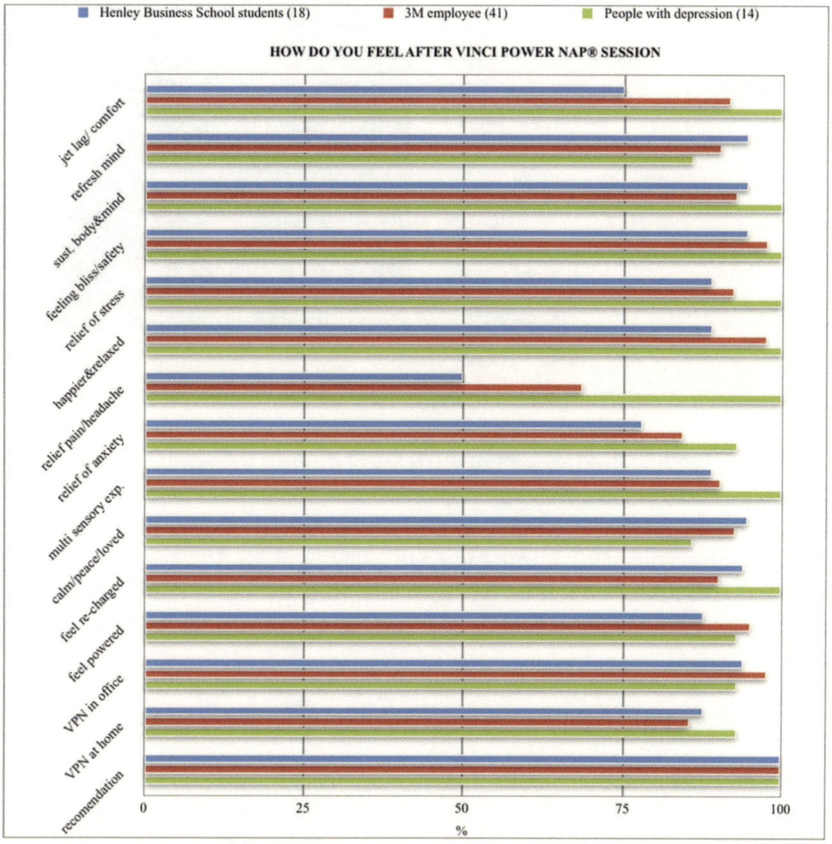


**Table 5.**
*Survey result levels of stress reductions after VPN sessions: Employees of 3 M company (41), BHS students (18), people with depression (14), source [40].*

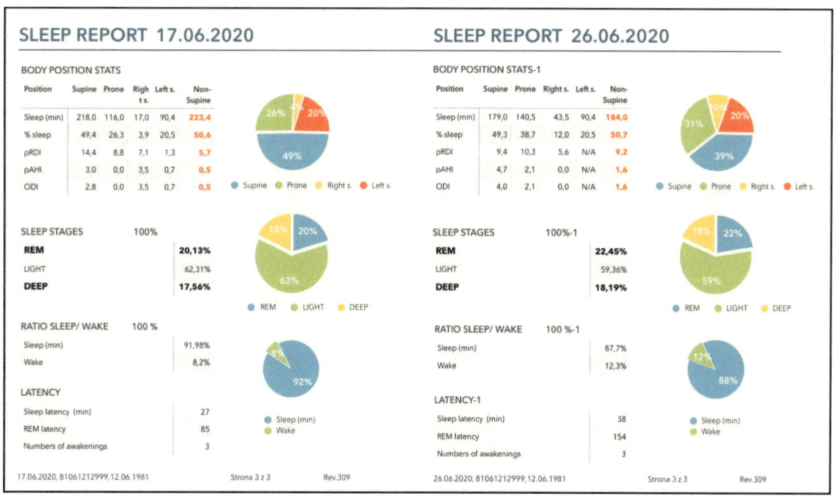

## SLEEP REPORT 17.06.2020

BODY POSITION STATS

| Position | Supine | Prone | Righ t s. | Left s. | Non-Supine |
|---|---|---|---|---|---|
| Sleep (min) | 218,0 | 116,0 | 17,0 | 90,4 | 223,4 |
| % sleep | 49,4 | 26,3 | 3,9 | 20,5 | 50,6 |
| pRDI | 14,4 | 8,8 | 7,1 | 1,3 | 5,7 |
| pAHI | 3,0 | 0,0 | 3,5 | 0,7 | 0,5 |
| ODI | 2,8 | 0,0 | 3,5 | 0,7 | 0,5 |



| SLEEP STAGES | 100% |
|---|---|
| **REM** | **20,13%** |
| LIGHT | 62,31% |
| **DEEP** | **17,56%** |



| RATIO SLEEP/ WAKE | 100 % |
|---|---|
| Sleep (min) | 91,98% |
| Wake | 8,2% |



| LATENCY | |
|---|---|
| Sleep latency (min) | 27 |
| REM latency | 85 |
| Numbers of awakenings | 3 |

17.06.2020, 81061212999,12.06.1981 Strona 3 z 3 Rev.309

## SLEEP REPORT 26.06.2020

BODY POSITION STATS-1

| Position | Supine | Prone | Right s. | Left s. | Non-Supine |
|---|---|---|---|---|---|
| Sleep (min) | 179,0 | 140,5 | 43,5 | 90,4 | 184,0 |
| % sleep | 49,3 | 38,7 | 12,0 | 20,5 | 50,7 |
| pRDI | 9,4 | 10,3 | 5,6 | N/A | 9,2 |
| pAHI | 4,7 | 2,1 | 0,0 | N/A | 1,6 |
| ODI | 4,0 | 2,1 | 0,0 | N/A | 1,6 |



| SLEEP STAGES | 100%-1 |
|---|---|
| **REM** | **22,45%** |
| LIGHT | 59,36% |
| **DEEP** | **18,19%** |



| RATIO SLEEP/ WAKE | 100 %-1 |
|---|---|
| Sleep (min) | 87,7% |
| Wake | 12,3% |



| LATENCY-1 | |
|---|---|
| Sleep latency (min) | 38 |
| REM latency | 154 |
| Numbers of awakenings | 3 |

26.06.2020, 81061212999,12.06.1981 Strona 3 z 3 Rev.309

**Figure 2.**
*Sleep report from polysonograph measurements of sleep on a soldier with PTSD during two nights, at the beginning and the end of 10 day VPN treatment.*

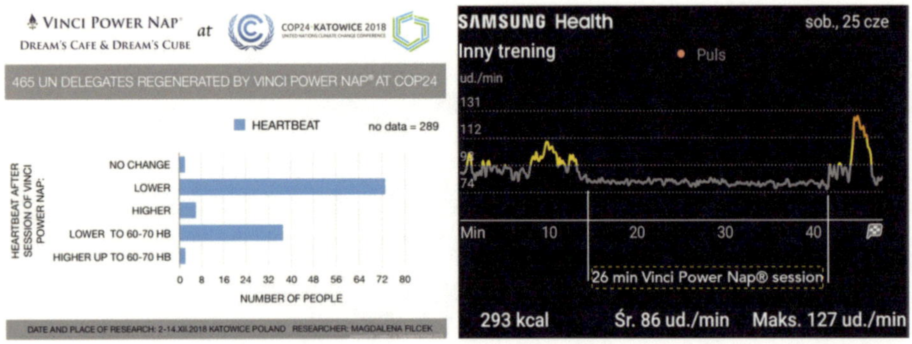


**Figure 3.**
*Heartbeat measurement of 176 UN delegates on COP24 [39] and end user.*

## 5.7 Experiment with reducing jet lag with VPN during Warsaw—Tokyo travel

The author experimented while traveling from Warsaw to Tokyo; shortly after landing, the author took a 20-minute nap while swinging in VPN cocoon. During the entire stay in Tokyo, she felt no jet lag at all, while the other conference attendees complained of severe time zone changing—jet lag symptoms throughout the whole week.

## 5.8 Feedback from top doctors in sleep medicine, scientists, and end users

Prof. P. Zimbardo—from Stanford University in California, USA—wrote that VPN allowed him for totally relax, deep sleep, and refresh energy; he is sure that this idea have to be translated into a global movement—which allows to help people in every age to unite heart, mind, spirit, and body. May 23, 2023 [124, 125].

Dr. M. Skalski, Specialist of Sleep Medicine and Sleep Disorders, Treatment Clinic and Warsaw Medical University, wrote that after the first VPN session, he let go of the physical and mental tensions, which made confirmation for his beliefs in this unique method—to achieve quick and deep relaxation. October 25, 2019 [124].

Dr. Mayank Vats, Senior Specialist, Intensivist, and Sleep Physician, Interventional Pulmonologist in Rashid Hospital and Dubai Health Authority in Dubai, UAE wrote in the letter to WHO and UN that as a COVID frontline warrior, he strongly recommend implementation Vinci Power Nap® system in every hospital to help reenergize the HCPs and reduce the physical and mental fatigue—it will allow them to work with fresh energy and efficiency. July 1, 2020 [124].

Dr. J. Lucas Koberda, MD, PhD., Neurologist at the Invisible Wound Center/ Intrepid Spirit Center/Eglin Air-force Base in Florida indicated that the Vinci Power Nap® could be potentially used as part of traumatic brain injury treatment. 10 June 2022 [124].

Director Mr. R. Juchniewicz—Head of the Pedagogical and Psychological Counseling Center of the Vilnius Region in Lithuania—wrote that after VPN session, he for the first time in many years felt calm, peace, deep relaxation, and rest after only 26 min. March 27, 2019 [124].

Dr. L. P. M. Klim from Bayer wrote that VPN is a great solution for any type of sleep disorder. July 7, 2020 [125].

ZEN Master Mr. A. Poraj—the creator of "Empty Cloud"—wrote that it is a great solution to take care of ourselves and rest—to be able help others. July 25, 2018 [125].

The owner of the Association of Space Relaxation Techniques wrote that VPN can give priceless feeling of withdrawal of the senses and regeneration on every level. January 10, 2019 [125].

Mrs. M. Maj—the mother of a child with sleep disorder—wrote that the VPN sleep therapy is working brilliantly. January10, 2023 [125].

Mrs. K. Majka wrote that VPN is a unique place where people can be reborn again, where mind and soul can become calmer. January 23, 2020 [125].

Mr. A. Kudelski, businessman from Zug, Switzerland, wrote that he feels that he was reborn after 20 min of VPN session and it was unique experience. August 7, 2022 [125].

Mr. Yuki Mitani, luxury taxi driver from Tokyo, wrote that it will be wonderful if VPN room could be implemented in a taxi company. June 11, 2019 [125].

NASA/JPL Flight Project Manager—Mr. A. Chmielewski—wrote that he trained many astronauts in his life, but he has never been on ISS, the space station; nevertheless during VPN session, he could feel how it is in space in zero gravity position. June 7, 2022 [125].

Mr. J. Skrzypczynski—top leaders' coach—wrote that in today's world, people are in rush, hurry, and stress, and for development, the most important is to relax; it is basic to have achievements in very field: in sports, work, medicine, learning, and even in making love. Vinci Power Nap® is a great tool for fast relaxation as benefit for yourself, your family, and colleagues. June 2, 2020 [125].

Ministry of Environment of Poland—Mr. M. Kurtyka wrote that 465 delegates of UN had the possibility to regenerate body and mind and achieve great success in negotiations during COP24, recommending this technology for conferences, trainings, and workshops. March 10, 2019 [124, 125].

Director Conference Affairs Services, United Nations Climate Change Secretariat, Mrs. L. Lopez wrote that VPN brought peaceful interlude during the hectic conference period and had great impact on people, recommending for other UN conferences in future. March 11, 2019 [124, 125].

And many more recommendations and feedbacks are in VPN Guest Books.

VPN system was presented all around the world on many top conferences—in subjects of sleep on "Sleep Expo" in Dubai in 2019, "Somnex" 2018 in London, a conference called "Smart Cities Powered by People" in New York in 2018, "Resilient and Responsible Architecture and Urbanism" in Malaysia 2019, "Future Smart Cities" in Kuala Lumpur 2020, and many more. VPN was presented as the great solution tool and help leaders, employees, shift workers, soldiers, drivers, pilots, astronauts, travelers, and others.

## 6. Conclusion

The author's pioneering interdisciplinary evidence-based research and end user feedbacks from thousands of hours of sessions confirm that Vinci Power Nap® neuroarchitecture system provides remarkable positive results in the reduction of fatigue, stress, and jet lag, allowing for synchronization of circadian rhythm, regeneration of body and mind, and increase in the well-being, quality of night's sleep, and energy for life. The VPN system-based discoveries empower understanding the relationship between environment stressors and the body's neurobiological reaction to them, which also triggers the release of histamine from mast cells, emphasizes the role of enzymes, as well as impacts these two on human psychophysical conditions related to inflammation, sleep, and emotions.

Vinci Power Nap® is a revolution system for balance and harmonization of: circulatory, respiratory, endocrine, lymphatic, and immune systems, has the ability to calm the brain waves and heart rhythm disorders (also tachycardia), and could help to restore homeostasis, increasing vitality and hormones oxytocin, serotonin, dopamine, testosterone, indirectly melatonin, and so on. All of this shows that VPN can be a wonderful tool using for prevention and as a help in the treatment for burnt-out, overtired, overwhelmed, depressed, traumatized, insomniac people; this innovation can also be helpful for people with Alzheimer's, Parkinson's disease, and so forth.

Vinci Power Nap®'s oscillation properties allow for synchronizing body rhythm systems, hydrodynamic pulsation accelerating enzymatic catalysis, and faster regeneration of damaged cells and their structure like increasing bone tissue density, which are also revolutionary findings for human space travels. VPN biological regulation functions have positive effect also for pilots and passengers of airplanes by helping to reduce stress, tiredness, and jet lag symptoms; recover sleep architecture; and improve cognitive/physical performance, focus, and efficiency.

Conclusions strongly highlight the need of implementation VPN solutions in the real world, for example, at travel-related facilities like hotels, airports, ships, spaceships, and Martian and Lunar habitats, as well as at hospitals, clinics, schools, trains, and so on; it will help to improve the well-being of travelers and inhabitants of future smart cities. Providing 20-min restorative power naps in innovative neuro-architecture allows for boosting energy during the day, memory, mental clarity, body regeneration, rejuvenation, and work–life balance and reducing stress, jet lag, risk of heart attacks, and so forth. VPN technology and its neurosensomotor stimulation is an exceptional form of napping in the right conditions, providing revolutionary tool to support sleep, well-being and health for decision-makers, leaders, employees, managers, students, surgeons, commanders, soldiers, pilots, astronauts, travelers in space, and all humankind on Earth. The author's suggestion is that VPN sessions and additional antihistamines H1 and H2; vitamins D3, C, B6; zinc; cooper; and the DAO enzyme before, during, and after space travels, long and fast journeys, may provide prevention and therapeutic effects and could also help to fall asleep faster and maintain a good night's sleep.

The interdisciplinary aspects of neurophysiological VPN system can help restore the mind–body connection; sleep and wake patterns in infants, children, adults, and seniors; and be applicable for fast restorative relaxation, prevention, and therapies, as well as bring a new perspective for future research with reference to sleep medicine, aviation and space medicine, interior design, neuroarchitecture, neuroscience, circadian rhythm, nervous systems, psychology, physiology, transplantology, molecular biology, embryology, longevity, harmonization of homeostasis, and other systems of human body.

## Conflict of interest

Magdalena Filcek, the author of the chapter, is also inventor of technology Vinci Power Nap® system.

## Author details

Magdalena Filcek[1*] and Mayank Vats[2,3,4]

1 Department Architecture of Interiors, Neuroarchitecture, Wroclaw, Poland

2 Pulmonology, Sleep Medicine, Dubai Hospital, Dubai Medical College, UAE

3 Interventional Pulmonologist and Critical care Medicine, Dubai Hospital, Dubai Medical College, UAE

4 Intensivist and Sleep Physician at Rashid Hospital, Dubai Hospital, Dubai Medical College, UAE

*Address all correspondence to: filcekmagdalena@gmail.com

## References

[1] Castanon-Cervantes O et al. Dysregulation of inflammatory responses by chronic circadian disruption. Journal of Immunology. 15 Nov 2010;**185**(10):5796-5805

[2] Cheung V et al. The effect of sleep deprivation and disruption on DNA damage and health of doctors. Anaesthesia. 2019;**74**(4):434-440

[3] Moldofsky H et al. Effects of sleep deprivation on human immune functions. The FASEB Journal. 1989;**3**(8):1972-1977

[4] Colten HR et al. Sleep Disorders and Sleep Deprivation: An Unmet Public Health Problem, 3Extent and Health Consequences of Chronic Sleep Loss and Sleep Disorders. Committee on Sleep Medicine and Research, National Acad. of Sciences; 2006

[5] Suni E, Truong K. 100+ Sleep Statistics. Sleep Foundation. 2022. Available from: https://www.sleepfoundation.org/how-sleep-works/sleep-factsstatistics

[6] Akerstedt T et al. Shift work and napping. In: Dinges DF, Broughton RJ, editors. Sleep and Alertness: Chronobiological, Behavioral and Medical Aspects of Napping. New York: Raven Press; 1989. pp. 205-220

[7] Fry A, Singh A. Coronasomnia: Definition, Symptoms, and Solutions. Sleep Foundation. 2023. Available from: https://www.sleepfoundation.org/covid-19-and-sleep/coronasomnia

[8] Watkins T. Researchers Urge Doctors to Disclose Sleep Fatigue before Surgery. CNN; 2010

[9] Locker M. The Scientific Secrets to Preventing Jet Lag. Time; 2018

[10] Sleep Foundation. Available from: https://www.sleepfoundation.org/ [Accessed: 2023-01-20]

[11] Matoso M. Neuroarchitecture: How your Brain Responds to Different Spaces. ArchDaily. 2022. Available from: https://www.archdaily.com/982248/neuroarchitecture-how-your-brainresponds-to-different-spaces

[12] Dr Cherry N. EMF/EMR Reduces Melatonin in Animals and People. New Zealand: Human Sciences Department Lincoln University Canterbury; 2002

[13] Huffington A. The Sleep Revolution: Transforming Your Life, One Night at a Time. Harmony Books. New York, NY: Crown Publishing Group and Penguin Random House LLC.; 2016. ISBN 978-1-101-90400-8

[14] Walker M. Why We Sleep. Scribner. 3 Oct 2017

[15] McCormick DA et al. Thalamocortical oscillations in the sleeping and aroused brain. Science. 1993;**262**(5134):679-685

[16] Kayaba M et al. Energy metabolism differs between sleep stages and begins to increase prior to awakening. Metabolism: Clinical and Experimental. 2017;**69**:14-23

[17] Liu Y et al. Prevalence of healthy sleep duration among adults—United States, 2014. MMWR. Morbidity and Mortality Weekly Report. 19 Feb 2016;**65**(6):137-141

[18] Bernardi G et al. Regional delta waves in human rapid eye movement sleep. Journal of Neuroscience. 3 Apr 2019;**39**(14):2686-2697

[19] Collins F. Discovering the Brain's Nightly "Rinse Cycle". 5 March 2020. Available from: https://directorsblog.nih.gov/2020/03/05/discovering-the-brains-nightly-rinse-cycle/

[20] Fultz NE et al. Coupled electrophysiological, hemodynamic, and cerebrospinal fluid oscillations in human sleep. Science. 1 Nov 2019;**366**(6465):628-631

[21] Jaekyung K et al. Competing roles of slow oscillations and delta waves in memory consolidation versus forgetting. Cell. 3 Oct 2019;**179**(2):283-578

[22] Carey B. Sleep therapy seem as an aid for depression. 2013. Available from: https://www.nytimes.com/2013/11/19/health/treating-insomnia-to-heal-depression.html. [Accessed: 2023-01-20]

[23] Khullar A. The role of melatonin in the circadian rhythm sleep-wake cycle. Psychiatric Times. 2012;**29**(7):2012

[24] Green A et al. Evening light exposure to computer screens disrupts human sleep, biological rhythms, and attention abilities. Chronobiology International. 2017;**34**(7):855-865

[25] Filcek M. Discovery of the Mechanism of COVID19, SIRS and SEPSIS, Defense and Treatment. Mast cells and Histamine Storm an Overlooked Aspects in COVID19 and in Ventilated Patients Potential Role of Antihistamine. MAR Pulmon.3.5

[26] Haas H et al. The role of histamine and the tuberomamillary nucleus in the nervous system. Nature Reviews. Neuroscience. 2003;**4**(2):121-130

[27] Butt AM et al. Effect of histamine and antagonists on electrical resistance across the blood-brain barrier in rat brain-surface microvessels. Brain Research. 8 Jan 1992;**569**(1)

[28] Fernandez-Novoa L et al. Histamine function in brain disorders. Behavioural Brain Research. 15 Oct 2001;**124**(2):213-233

[29] Nuutinen S et al. Histamine in Neurotransmission and Brain Diseases. In: Histamine in Inflamation. Springer. 2010

[30] Karpati A. et al. Histamine elicits glutamate release from cultured astrocytes. Journal of Pharmacological Science. Jun 2018;**137**(2):122-128

[31] Ebrahim IO et al. Alcohol and sleep I: Effects on normal sleep. Alcoholism: Clinical and Experimental Research. Apr 2013;**37**(4):539-549

[32] Garcia AN et al. Polysomnographic sleep disturbances in nicotine, caffeine, alcohol, cocaine, opioid, and cannabis use: A focused review. The American Journal on Addictions. Oct 2015;**24**(7):590-598

[33] Okamoto-Mizuno K et al. Effects of thermal environment on sleep and circadian rhythm. Journal of Physiological Anthropology. 2012;**31**(1):14

[34] Cherry K. Deep Sleep and the Impact of Delta Waves. 6 October 2021

[35] Abbas AB et al. Innate immunity. In: Basic Immunology. Functions and Disorders of the Immune System. 3rd ed. Saunders (Elsevier); 2009

[36] St-Onge M-P et al. Effects of diet on sleep quality. Advances in Nutrition. Sep 2016;**7**(5):938-949

[37] Edlund MJ. Want to Treat Depression? Get People to Sleep. Fix

insomnia and better things happen. 21 November 2013. Available from: https://www.psychologytoday.com/us/blog/the-power-rest/201311/want-treat-depression-get-people-sleep [Accessed: 2023-01-20]

[38] Soojung-Kim PA. Rest–Why You Get More Done When You Work less. Penguin Books Ltd. 16 Jul 2018. ISBN: 9780241217290

[39] Filcek M. Innovative Vinci Power Nap® neurotechnology system—to reset and reconnect the senses, body and mind; reducing stress, improving performance, sleep, health and quality of life. In: Resilient and Responsible Smart Cities. Springer. 2022. pp. 249-264

[40] Filcek M. The neuroarchitecture technology of Vinci Power Nap: A revolution in fast stress reduction, newborns protection, well-being and sleep regeneration also for people with trauma, depression and PTSD in smart cities. Journal of Psychiatry and Psychiatric Disorders. 2022;**6**(2):61-104

[41] Sleep Education Archive. Sleep in the city: big-city living may cause insomnia, sleep loss. 2008. Retrieved November 12, 2020. Available from: http://sleepeducation.org/news/2008/09/26/sleep-in-the-city-big-city-living-may-cause-insomnia-sleep-loss

[42] Stevenson S. Sleep Smarter: 21 Essential Strategies to Sleep Your Way to a Better Body, Better Health, and Bigger Success. United Kingdom: HAY House; 2016

[43] Zhao D. et al. Melatonin Synthesis and Function: Evolutionary History in Animals and Plants. 2019

[44] The Pineal Gland and Melatonin. VIVO Pathophysiology, Pathophysiology of the Endocrine System, Fundamental Concepts in Endocrinology; Nov 2018. Available from: http://www.vivo.colostate.edu/hbooks/pathphys/endocrine/otherendo/pineal.html

[45] Xie Z et al. A review of sleep disorders and melatonin. Neurological Research. Jun 2017;**39**(6):559-565

[46] Mottolese R et al. Switching Brain Serotonin with Oxytocin. In: Leslie GU, editor. Proceedings of the National Academy of Sciences of the United States of America. Biological Science. Bethesda, MD: National Institute of Mental Health; 29 Apr 2014

[47] Suofu V et al. Dual role of mitochondria in producing melatonin and driving GPCR signaling to block cytochrome c release. Proceedings of the National Academy of Sciences of the United States of America. 19 Sep 2017;**114**(38):E7997-E8006

[48] Ketchum A. The More you Hug your Kids, the More their Brains Develop. 2019 Baby Chick. Parenting; Jul 21 2023. Available from: https://www.baby-chick.com/themore-you-hug-your-kids-the-moretheir-brains-develop/

[49] Sohal VS. Serotonin gives oxytocin a helping hand. Science Translational Medicine. 16 Oct 2013;**5**(207):207ec172

[50] Tsai LL et al. Repeated light-dark shifts speed up body weight gain in male f344 rats. American Journal of Physiology. Endocrinology and Metabolism. Aug 2005;**289**(2):E212-E217

[51] Gardner MJ et al. How plants tell the time. The Biochemical Journal. 1 Jul 2006;**397**(Pt 1):15-24

[52] Tan DX et al. Melatonin: A hormone, a tissue factor, an autocoid, a paracoid, and an antioxidant vitamin. Journal of Pineal Research. Jan 2003;**34**(1):75-78

[53] Yoo SH. et al. Period2::Luciferase real-time reporting of circadian dynamics reveals persistent circadian oscillations in mouse peripheral tissues. PNAS. Biological Sciences. 12 Feb 2004;**101**(15):5339-5346

[54] Yamazaki S et al. Resetting central and peripheral circadian oscillators in transgenic rats. Science. 28 Apr 2000;**288**(5466):682-685

[55] Gamble KL et al. Circadian clock control of endocrine factors. Nature Reviews. Endocrinology. Aug 2014;**10**(8):466-475

[56] Cambras T et al. Circadian desynchronization of core body temperature and sleep stages in the rat. Proceedings of the National Academy of Sciences of the United States of America. 1 May 2007;**104**(18):7634-7639

[57] Filcek M. Frequency of harmony and the unified theory of everything. Across the Universe towards Human Body and Mind with Discovery of Neuroarchitecture Vinci Power Nap® Pendulum as the Biotechnology of the Future. Journal of Biotechnology and Biomedicine. 2022

[58] Fiedorowicz A. et al. Drzemka za biurkiem? Pracodawca powinien je zalecać. 2018. Available from: https://www.focus.pl/artykul/drzemka-za-biurkiem. [Accessed: 2023-01-20]

[59] Howell E. Weightlessness and its effect on astronauts. 2017. Available from: https://www.space.com/23017-weightlessness.html [Accessed: 2023-01-20]

[60] Littlehales N. Sleep: Redefine Your Rest, for Success in Work, Sport and Life. Penguin Life; 2016. ISBN 10: 0241975972

[61] Powell A. Sleeping your Way to Heart Health. A Nap a Day May Keep the Cardiologist Away, Study Finds. The Harvard Gazette; 15 February 2007. Available from: https://news.harvard.edu/gazette/story/2007/02/sleeping-your-way-to-heart-health/

[62] Liao S et al. Lymphatic function and immune regulation in health and disease. Lymphatic Research and Biology. Sep 2013;**11**(3):136-143

[63] Gardner EP. Touch. New York University School of Medicine. 2010. Available from: https://www.cns. nyu.edu/*david/courses/sm12/Readings/Gardner-ELS2010.pdf

[64] Viens A. Global Health. Are you Sleeping Enough? This Infographic Shows How you Compare to the Rest of the World. 16 Aug 2019. Available from: https://www.weforum.org/agenda/2019/08/we-need-more-sleep

[65] Hongzhong L et al. The allergy mediator histamine confers resistance to immunotherapy in cancer patients via activation of the macrophage histamine receptor H1. Cancer Cell. 2022;**40**(1):36-52. E9

[66] Porges S. The polyvagal theory: New insights into adaptive reactions of the autonomic nervous system. Cleveland Clinic Journal of Medicine. Apr 2009:**76**(Suppl. 2):S86-S90

[67] 9 Fascinating facts about the Vagus nerve. 12 April 2021. Available from: https://www.mentalfloss.com/article/65710/9-nervy-facts-about-vagus-nerve?fbclid=IwAR0QJ6wkYo3HKMDnMpPnlrD0QVpwuacFKVwIiG1S1O5uaCEQC2P6DHbNqrE

[68] Filcek M. Cutting edge solution for effective and safe missions - neuroarchitecture system of Vinci

power nap® - revolution in fast stress reduction, regeneration, regenerating body and mind, which can help you, pilots, astronauts: Before, during and after space travels. In: 71st International Astronautical Congress 2020. 2020. Available from: https://dl.iafastro.directory/event/IAC-2020/paper/56737/

[69] Martín-Alguacil N et al. Somatosensation: End organs for tactile sensation. In: Pfaff DW, editor. Neuroscience in the 21st Century. New York, NY: Springer; 2013

[70] Deli MA. Histamine and the blood-brain barrier. In: Histamine: Biology and Medical Aspects. Karger; 2004

[71] The lymphatic system how to improve it natural recommendations. Natural Ways of Lymphangitis. 1932

[72] Re:Re. The Glymphatic System - CSF와 림프액의 순환. 20 June 2020. Available from: https://m.cafe.daum.net/panicbird/OU8N/164. [Accessed: 2023-01-20]

[73] Alstadhaug KB. Histamine in migraine and brain. Headache. The Journal of Head and Face Pain. 16 Jan 2014;**54**(2):246-259

[74] Tripathi AK et al. Acceleration of enzymatic catalysis by active hydrodynamic fluctuations. Communications on Physics. 2022;**5**:10

[75] Richard HW et al. Effects of Electromagnetic Fields on Cells: Physiological and Therapeutical Approaches and Molecular Mechanisms of Interaction a Review. Dep. of Anatomy, University of Technology, Dresden, Germany Cells Tissues Organs; 2006

[76] Rand DA et al. Uncovering the design principles of circadian clocks: Mathematical analysis of flexibility and evolutionary goals. Journal of Theoretical Biology. 7 Feb 2006;**238**(3):616-635

[77] Dodd AN et al. Plant circadian clocks increase photosynthesis, growth, survival, and competitive advantage. Science. 2005;**309**:630-633

[78] Eastman CI et al. How to Travel the World without Jet Lag. Sleep Medicine Clinics. 1 Jun 2009;**4**(2):241-255

[79] Bin YS et al. What works for jetlag? A systematic review of non-pharmacological interventions. Sleep Medicine Reviews. Feb 2019;**43**:47-59

[80] Cingi C et al. Jetlag Related Sleep Problems and their Management. Travel Medicine and Infectious Disease. Jul-Aug 2018;**24**:59-64

[81] Sack RL. The pathophysiology of jet lag. Travel Medicine and Infectious Disease. Mar 2009;**7**(2):102-110

[82] American Academy of Sleep Medicine. AASM sets standards and promotes excellence in sleep medicine health care, education, and research. Available from: https://aasm.org/

[83] Golombek DA et al. Minutes, days and years: Molecular interactions among different scales of biological timing. Philosophical Transactions of the Royal Society of London. Series B, Biological Sciences. 5 Mar 2014;**369**(1637):20120465

[84] Bragazzi NL et al. Planetary sleep medicine: Studying sleep at the individual, population, and planetary level. Frontiers in Public Health. 2022;**10**:1005100

[85] El-Esawi MA. Circadian Rhythms and their Molecular Mechanisms. London, UK: IntechOpen; 2018

[86] Collins B et al. Keeping time without a clock. 4 May 2006;**50**(3):348-350

[87] Michinaga S et al. Selective histamine $H_2$ receptor agonists alleviate blood-brain barrier disruption by promoting the expression of vascular protective factors following traumatic brain injury in mice. Journal of Pharmacological Sciences. 3 Nov 2022;**150**(3)

[88] Vosko AM et al. Jet lag syndrome: Circadian organization, pathophysiology, and management strategies. Nature and Science of Sleep. 19 Aug 2010;**2**:187-198

[89] Dijk DJ et al. Sleep, circadian rhythms, and performance during space shuttle missions. The Neurolab Spacelab Mission: Neuroscience Research in Space: Results from the STS-90 Neurolab Spacelab Mission. NASA- SP 2003-353. 2013

[90] Buxton OM et al. Sleep disruption due to hospital noises. 7 August 2012

[91] Boyle R et al. Challenges to the central nervous system during human spaceflight missions to Mars. Advances in Vestibular Research: A Tribute to Bernard Cohen. Journal of Neurophysiology. May 2020;**123**(5):2037-2063

[92] Chu J. MIT Engineers Fly First-Ever Plane with no Moving Parts. The Silent, Lightweight Aircraft doesn't Depend on Fossil Fuels. MIT NEWS; 21 Nov 2018. Available from: https://news.mit.edu/2018/first-ionic-wind-plane-no-moving-parts-1121

[93] DeBaun DT. Ways to reduce EMF exposure while flying in an airplane. EMF Protection & Safety, Travel. 2019 updated 13 May 2022 by Daniel T. DeBaun: Engineer, Author & Telecommunications Executive 7 Aug 2019. Available from: https://defendershield.com/doesflying-airplane-increase-emfradiation-exposure

[94] #PowiedzSprawdzam: Raki w samolocie. Available from: https://www.gov.pl/web/5g/powiedzsprawdzam-raki-w-samolocie. [Accessed: 2023-01-20]

[95] Stratton D et al. Extremely low-frequency magnetic fields significantly enhance the cytotoxicity of methotrexate and can reduce migration of cancer cell lines via transiently induced plasma membrane damage. Biochemical and Biophysical Research Communications. 2022;**626**:192-199

[96] Indii. Szkodliwe skutki promieniowania elektromagnetycznego i pól elektromagnetycznych. 11 Octob 2016. Available from: https://sklep.qtherm.pl/pl/n/34

[97] Zablotskii et al. How a high-gradient magnetic field could affect cell life. Scientific Reports. 2016;**6**:37407

[98] Goldstein DS. Stress-induced activation of the sympathetic nervous system. Bailliere's Clinical Endocrinology and Metabolism. 1987;**1**(2):253-278

[99] NASA Human Research Program. Risk of performance decrements and adverse health outcomes resulting from sleep loss. Circadian Desynchronization, and Work Overload. Human Research Program Behavioral Health and Performance Element Approved for Public Release: National Aeronautics and Space Administration Lyndon B. Johnson Space Center Houston, Texas. Apr 11 2016. Available from: https://humanresearchroadmap.nasa.gov/evidence/reports/sleep.pdf

[100] van Dongen HPA, et al. The cumulative cost of additional wakefulness: Dose-response effects on

neurobehavioral functions and sleep physiology from chronic sleep restriction and total sleep deprivation. Sleep. Journal of Sleep and Sleep Disorders Research. 2003;**26**(2):117-126

[101] Sleep Oscillations in Space. 29 Aug 2019. Available from: https://www.esa.int/gsp/ACT/projects/sleep_oscillations_in_space/. [Accessed: 2023-01-20]

[102] Fatigue Management Guide for Airplane Operators. II ed. Airlines magazine. The International Air Transport Association (IATA). 2015. Available from: https://www.iata.org/contentassets/39bb2b7d6d5b40c6abf88c11111fcd12/fatigue-managementguide_airline20operators.pdf [Accessed: January 20, 2023]

[103] Flight crew Fatigue Recommendations for airlines on reducing and preventing crew fatigue. Delft University of Technology Faculty of Technology, Policy and Management Safety Science Group Raymond Dijkshoorn Student number: 9211477. 2008

[104] Dacey J. Yawning drivers urged to power nap. 11 March 2011. Available from: https://www.swissinfo.ch/eng/yawning-drivers-urged-to-power-nap/29695114

[105] Huffington A. Take the Pledge to Not Drive Drowsy. #TakeABreakToStayAwake change.org. Available from: https://www.change.org/p/take-the-pledge-to-not-drive-drowsy-takeabreaktostayawake

[106] Kauffman L. On the road to fewer fatigue crashes. Commercial Transportation. Sleep Review. 2015. Available from: https://sleepreviewmag.com/practice-management/lawsregulations/commercialtransportation/road-fewer-fatiguecrashes-mark-r-rosekind-phd-nhtsa/

[107] Young JA. The Effects of Life-Stress on Pilot Performance. NASA/TM-2008-215375. National Aeronautics and Space Administration. Moffett Field, California: Ames Research Center. 2008

[108] Rosekind MR et al. Factors in Flight Operations IX: Effects of Planned Cockpit Rest on Crew Performance and Alertness in Long-Haul Operations (NASA Technical Memorandum 108839). California: NASA Ames Research Center; 1994

[109] Rosekind MR et al. Alertness management: Strategic naps in operational settings. Journal of Sleep Research. Dec 1995;**4**(S2):62-66

[110] Rosekind MR et al. Alertness management in aviation operations: Enhancing performance and sleep. Aviation, Space, and Environmental Medicine. Dec 2006;77(12):1256-1265(10)

[111] Selby B, et al. NASA helps pilots combat fatigue during long flights. 2014. Available from: https://www.nasa.gov/home/hqnews/1994/94-177.txt. [Accessed: 2023-01-20]

[112] Stanford University. The Facts of Napping. Stanfordsdprod. 2013. Available from: https://youtu.be/vAETBvjl4gQ

[113] Stein L. Napping may be good for your heart. Scientific American. 12 Feb 2017. Available from: https://www.scientificamerican.com/article/napping-good-for-heart/

[114] Clément G. Fundamentals of Space Medicine. Springer; 2011

[115] Kanas N et al. Space Psychology and Psychiatry. The book Springer. 2008

[116] Tambala NJ. Fatigue on the flight deck. In: Challenges & Mitigations Concerning Fatigue in the Norwegian Aviation Sector. IE&TM; June 2017

[117] Williams K. NASA Research Reveals Biological Clock Misalignment Effects on Sleep for Astronauts. Ames Research Center; 7 Jan 2016

[118] NASA JPL Recommendations for Vinci Power Nap® from Artur Chmielewski, Menager NASA JPL. Available from: https://vincipowernap.asysto.pl/strona/8791-nasa-jpl-recommendation

[119] Szymański L. Wpływ fal elektromagnetycznych na organizmy. 5G Centrum Kompetencji Polytechnic Lodz. Available from: https://centrumkompetencji5g.pl/index.php/home/11-sample-articles/39-demo-article-2

[120] Beh SF et al. Air travelers' experiences and understanding of jetlag and perceptions of management strategies: A qualitative study. Ergonomics. Apr 2022;**65**(4):642-658

[121] Tan Z et al. Advances in the clinical application of histamine and diamine oxidase (DAO). Activity: A Review. Catalysts. 2023;**13**(1):48

[122] Perski A. The Book: Stress. Kielce: Poradnik na trudne czasy; 2022

[123] Shah P et al. Travel and sleep. American Thoracic Society. American Journal of Respiratory and Critical Care Medicine. American Journal of Respiratory and Critical Care Medicine ATS Patient Education Series © 2021 American Thoracic Society. 2021;**203**:P1-P2. Available from: https://www.thoracic.org/patients/patient-resources/resources/travel-and-sleep.pdf

[124] Recommendations for Vinci Power Nap® from UN, UNICEF, NASA, Polish and US ARMY, Professors, Doctors, etc. Available from: https://vincipowernap.asysto.pl/strona/8346-recommendation. [Accessed: January 20, 2023]

[125] Filcek M. Vinci Power Nap® synchronization technology - Neuroarchitecture for better sleep, adding energy for life, reducing stress and jet lag, improving wellbeing and body-mind regeneration. Helpful for leaders, doctors, soldiers, children, drivers, pilots, astronauts, people traveling on earth and beyond. Journal of Biotechnology and Biomedicine. 2023;**6**:105-128